To Ed & Kay Lester
Best regards
Carl Schlicke

—WORKING TOGETHER—

* * *

A HISTORY OF A MEDICAL GROUP PRACTICE

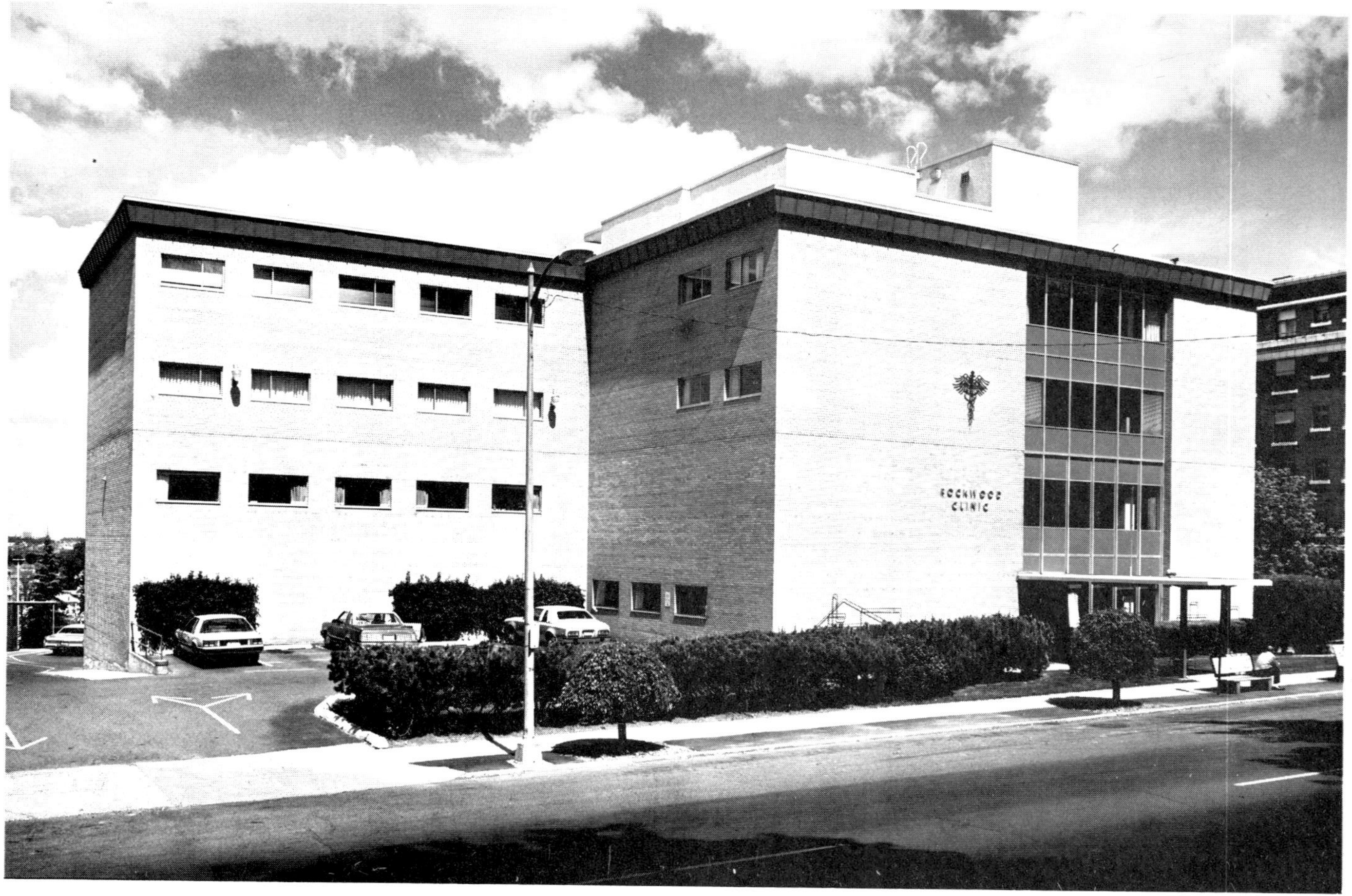

Present Rockwood Clinic Building

WORKING TOGETHER

A HISTORY *of a* MEDICAL GROUP PRACTICE, *THE ROCKWOOD CLINIC*

SPOKANE, WASHINGTON

CARL P. SCHLICKE, M.D.

YE GALLEON PRESS
FAIRFIELD, WASHINGTON
1980

The views and opinions expressed in this book are those of the author and do not necessarily reflect the views of the Rockwood Clinic or its partners.

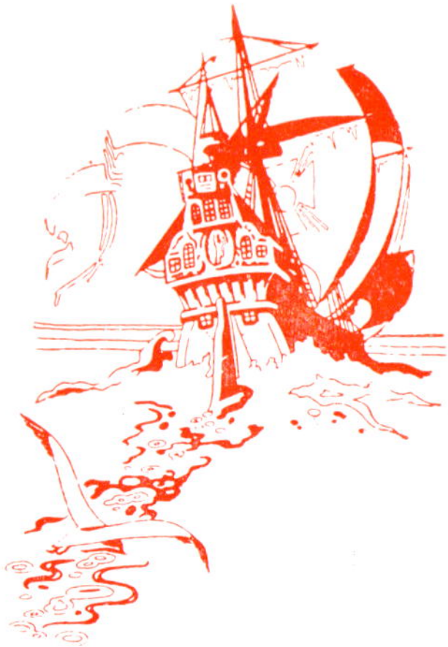

Library of Congress Cataloging in Publication Data

Schlicke, Carl Paul, 1910-
Working Together.

Includes index.
1. Rockwood Clinic—History. I. Title.
RA982.S78R627 362.1'2'0979737 80-21598
ISBN 0-87770-238-1

To all those fine people with whom it has been my privilege to spend my professional life—the doctors and staff of the Rockwood Clinic.

"What is human life without some purpose or end which may be attained by industry, order and exercise of moderate abilities? Great abilities are rare and often accompanied by qualities which make the abilities useless to him who has them and even injurious to society."

CONTENTS

ILLUSTRATIONS

PREFACE

ANYONE ATTEMPTING TO COMPILE a History of the Rockwood Clinic is immediately confronted with two major obstacles. The first is the paucity of records pertaining to the operation of the original Clinic prior to World War Two. The second is the difficulty of presenting an account of the present Clinic without duplicating or at least plagiarizing the product of Arch Jenkins' facile pen, "The Roots of Rockwood." Every effort has been made to avoid doing this but since both authors have drawn on much of the same source material, namely the minutes of the Rockwood Clinic Partnership, Holding Corporation and Foundation and a newspaper clipping album certain similarities are inevitable. Discrepancies in dates may be due to differences in the time events were recorded by the three Clinic entities. Minute reading, usually a dull pastime, has had its rewarding moments when Jenkins' characteristic touch and sense of humor showed through. Surprisingly, momentous events which occurred beyond their immediate scope never found their way into the minutes.

Inaccuracies will no doubt appear since much of the material concerning the pre-war years has been culled from the memories of those who lived through them. Portions of the account must inevitably assume an autobiographical cast but an earnest attempt has been made to keep these at a minimum. Every effort has been exerted to ascertain and present the facts as accurately as possible and to avoid passing judgement and editorializing, leaving it to the reader to draw his own conclusions.

It may seem strange in an account of a medical organization that so little is said of the main purpose of the group's existence, the patient. However, this is a narrative of the attempt by a number of individuals to develop and carry on a cooperative enterprise in the hope of offering better service to the individual patient. It is an account of the problems encountered, relationships within and outside of the group and the outcome up to the present. The Clinic sought to attract high caliber physicians and expected them to devote the major portion of their efforts, to the best of each individual's ability, to patient care. There were no great scholars, a few competent investigators, but they were all dedicated men who spent a great many more hours in the care of the sick and injured than the later official four and a half day work week would suggest. Some attained honors and recognition, some contributed generously of their time to political and public service projects, others developed fascinating avocations. For the most part they were happy, worked well together and liked and respected each other.

Additional information about the old Clinic has come from the Spokane Public Library, Newspaper files, Spokane County Medical Society records and the microfilm section in the Clerk of the Court's office. The surviving members of the pre-war group, Drs. Harold T. Pederson, Roy C. Biehn and Francis M. Lyle have been generous in supplying information. Others who have been most helpful have been Tod and Vera Oien, Grethe Henshaw, Mrs. A.R. Merman, Otto Warn and Vesta R. Prather. Particular thanks are due to some of the remaining members of Dr. W.W. Robinson's family: Mrs. Cecil P. Lyon, Mrs. Lyle R. Bain, Mrs. Edward P. Coleman, and Mrs. Betty O'Neal. Special gratitude is owing to one who has suffered much and been a great help, Mrs. Elsie P. Crawford. Appreciation is expressed to Mrs. Irene Qualtieri for her untiring efforts and support and for the typing of this manuscript.

But from whatever source, the piecing together of these fragments has resulted in a story not entirely devoid of interest, a story which hopefully will give the reader a better understanding of the growth, development, organization, management and underlying philosophy of the Rockwood Clinic of 1980. By a coincidence the compilation of this material has been completed just fifty years after the opening of the original Rockwood Clinic and its hospital.

To my partners, who insisted that this history be written and for whom it is chiefly intended, I can only express my thanks for their tolerance of my foibles and for the warm friendships I have enjoyed through all these years.

Carl P. Schlicke, M.D.

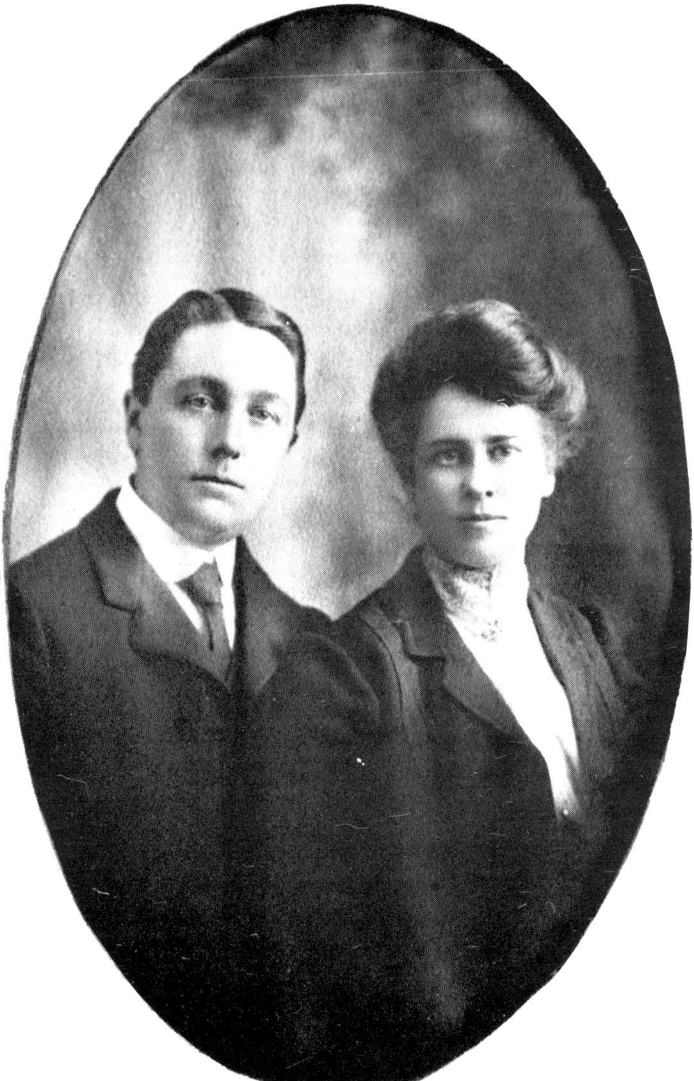

Fig. 1. Dr. and Mrs. Lesco A. Robinson
1904

1

THE MUSICAL FAMILY ROBINSON

AS IS SO OFTEN EXPLAINED to patients and visitors, the Rockwood Clinic did not derive its name from a legendary Doctor Rockwood. It refers to a district called Rockwood on the South Hill of Spokane, Washington, an area distinguished by its lofty ponderosa pines and its basaltic outcroppings, on the north edge of which the original Rockwood Clinic was located. There was, however, very definitely a founder, a colorful and controversial individual named William Witten Robinson.

W.W. Robinson was born in Glenwood Springs, Colorado in 1897. It was here that his father, Lesco A. Robinson, met, wooed and married Pamelia Eleanor Witten. (Fig. 1) She had come to Glenwood Springs to visit her father who had moved there from the ancestral home in Virginia. Lesco at this time was an impoverished druggist who after his marriage decided he wanted to become a doctor. He worked hard, struggled and saved and was admitted to Rush Medical College. His wife worked in a millinery store and he in a pharmacy to help make ends meet. Their first child, Bonnie, was born while they were in Chicago. Lesco received his M.D. degree in 1896 and they moved back to Glenwood Springs where he started his practice as an old fashioned, horse and buggy general practitioner. The next four children were born there, William (Bill), Gilbert Phillip (Bob), Eleanor and Dorothy (Dode). Dr. Robinson's practice grew rapidly but he was a very religious man and decided that a small resort town with its saloons and gambling was no place to raise a family.

Leaving the rest of the children in Glenwood Springs, Lesco and Pamelia, taking with them their youngest child, went on a tour of the Northwest and California in 1904, seeking a new location. They finally decided on Spokane as their future home and in 1907, after the birth of another child, Catherine (Tine), the whole family moved there, bringing with them Pamelia's father, a Confederate veteran of the Civil War. Lesco purchased two lots at 1025 West Cleveland and rented a little house across the street while the family home and an adjacent office were being built. Once established there, Lesco practiced medicine and surgery in Spokane until his death in 1935.

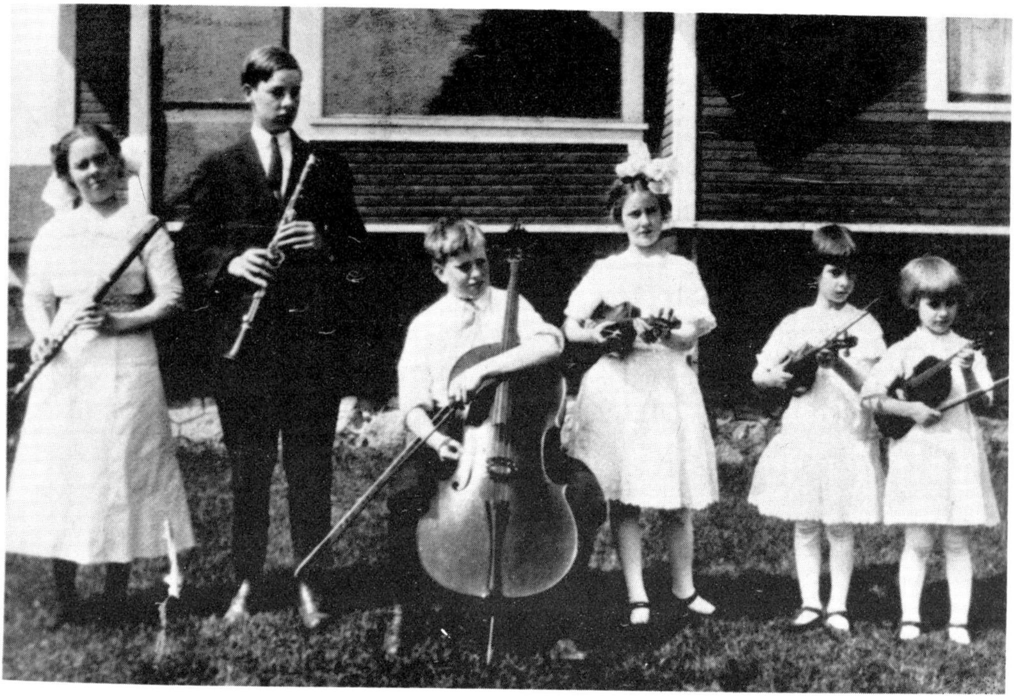

Fig. 2. The Robinson Family Orchestra, 1911
Bonnie, Bill, Bob, Eleanor, Dorothy, Catherine

WORKING TOGETHER

There was a new baby every two years or so, eleven in all, seven girls and four boys. According to Dode, "We had a happy childhood, not much money but lots of love and concern for each. We all attended Emerson Grade School, then on to the North Central High School. Seven of us attended Washington State College in Pullman." It was Lesco's dream to establish a Robinson Clinic. Although three of his sons became physicians and two of his daughters registered nurses his dream of a family clinic was never realized.

Dode tells how the older children used to take turns assisting their father in his small surgery next to their home, even giving drop ether anesthesia for such procedures as tonsillectomies and other "minor operations", and cleaning and sterilizing instruments. Fortunately no disasters occurred. Much of the children's play even was geared to medicine.

Pamelia, the mother, was an excellent pianist and saw to it that the children had music lessons—Bonnie on the flute, Bill, the clarinet, Bob the cello and the next three girls the violin. A family orchestra was formed with Mrs. Robinson playing the piano. (Fig. 2) There is even said to have been a drummer at one time but his percussions tended to drown out the musical efforts of the others so he was discouraged from further participation. In a short time the musical group became good enough to play out in public and made many appearances for various functions in Spokane. After one of the concerts Lesco was asked if he played an instrument. "Only the purse," he replied. However, he enjoyed the music and took pride in the family performances.

"Papa," as the children called him, was quite an individualist. During a period of economic depression he heard of some of his patients putting off seeing a doctor because they could not afford to pay. Feeling that everyone who needed medical attention should have it whether they could pay or not, he had a large sign made which said in effect, "Free treatment every Thursday for those needing medical care who cannot afford to pay." This he placed in the yard in front of his office. Although some people may have taken advantage of him, most showed deep gratitude—"EXCEPT [Dode's capitals] the County Medical Society." He received a severe reprimand for advertising and unprofessional conduct, however, he continued his charity "acting according to his faith and conscience." For his services he would accept payments of all types and the family would get "hair cuts, boxes of apples, potatoes, wood for the fireplace, even shoe

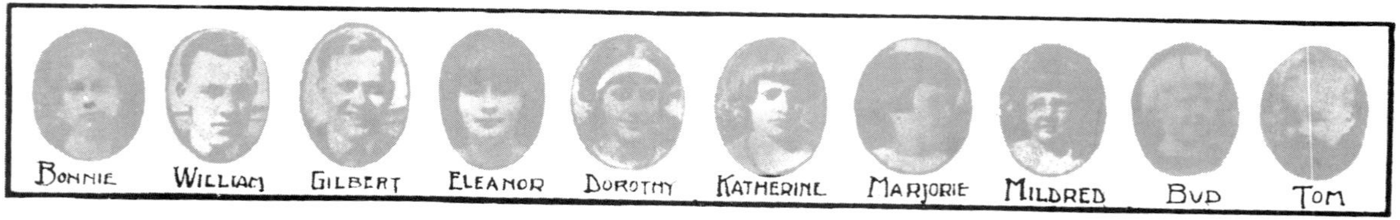

"WHY I NEED THE MONEY"

Spokane, Washington, ______________ 191

M ______________________________

To L. A. Robinson, M. D., Dr.

1025 CLEVELAND AVENUE

PHONE MAXWELL 3196

To Professional Services Rendered, $ ______________

By Cash, $ ______________

Balance, $ ______________

Fig. 3. One of Dr. L.A. Robinson's Bill-heads

repair on the doctor bill. A far cry from Medicare, Welfare, etc.," Dode observes.

At one stage of his career Lesco sent out some imaginative statements for his professional services. It turns out that these were a birthday present from Pamelia who had had young William take snapshots of the ten children living at that time and had them made into bill-heads with one of several captions underneath, "My ten reasons for cash," "Why I need the money," and "Ten strong reasons for cash." (Fig. 3) These were at first a source of embarrassment to the older children but later grudgingly accepted. Their use was short-lived, however, since little Marjorie died the next year so they were never used again. The children were very close to their father who loved them dearly but with the exception of Bill were rather aloof from their mother who seems at times to have had some severe emotional problems.

The oldest child, Bonnie, graduated from the Deaconess Hospital School of Nursing. She worked there for a few years and then married the son of an old Glenwood Springs friend. She and her husband moved back to Glenwood Springs. It is said that her married life was unhappy and ended in a divorce; she later died from cancer.

Bill, the next child, was two years younger. His sister, Dode, said, "As a youngster he showed an intense interest in everything medical and scientific. He collected insects of every variety he could find, and mounted them neatly on pins in cigar boxes in his room. Woe be it to anyone who dared to disturb them! He had an old microscope with which he studied the various frogs and polliwogs he had dissected." When the children engaged in medical play, Bill was always the surgeon, Bob his assistant and the girls nurses. "He built a glider from plans he found in Popular Mechanics, that he planned on flying off Monroe Hill, but finding severe disapproval from Papa, sold it to one of his friends who promptly tried to fly in it and broke both legs. Rather than cranking the handle of our old ice cream freezer, he jacked up the rear end of our old Overland car, rigged the wheel to the handle, and froze the ice cream so hard it broke the dasher." More of Bill later.

Bob, after taking his premedical work at Washington State College earned an M.D. degree at Loyola University. He was an accomplished cellist and while in Chicago played in a trio which provided dinner music at one of that city's finer restaurants. He interned at Los Angeles County Hospital. In the meanwhile he married his first cousin, Louise Witten, the daughter of Pamelia's brother, Thomas. After his internship, he and his wife and their one year old son, Tom, returned to Spokane where he went into practice with his father, Lesco, in July, 1929. That December after a bad flu epidemic, during which he had been going night and day on house calls, he became ill himself. He developed meningitis and died three days later on Christmas Day, at St. Luke's Hospital, a few days before his thirtieth birthday. His son, Thomas Witten Robinson, went into medicine and is a practicing pediatrician in Newport Beach, California. Eleanor attended Washington State for two years, was married for a short time, and eventually took up nurse's training at Good Samaritan Hospital in Los Angeles. Somewhere along the line she had a "nervous breakdown" and had to be institutionalized. She later did very well, received many promotions and eventually became Superintendent of Nurses at the Good Samaritan Hospital. She is now deceased.

Dorothy was the first of the children to depart from the field of medicine. She graduated from Washington State College (WSC) in music, a violin major. She had joined the Spokane Musicians' Union at fifteen and began playing professionally at that time. She studied violin at the Chicago Conservatory for a year while Bill and Bob were in Chicago. After graduation she went to Portland where she played with the Portland Symphony Orchestra and at radio station KOIN for seven years. Her second year in Portland "Dode" married Lyle Bain, a second year student at the University of Oregon Medical School. After graduation her husband interned at Multnomah County Hospital and then they moved to his home town of Albany, Oregon, where he set up in general practice. As a member of the Oregon National Guard, Lyle was activated in 1940 and spent five years in the South Pacific. He was never quite well after his long stay in the tropics but lived until 1973 when he passed away after seven years of blindness. Dode ultimately had to give up the violin because of a shoulder problem but took up the organ which she plays for style shows and other events. She is still living in Albany and has one son, Bill, and three grandchildren in Eugene.

Catherine married a veterinarian after two years at WSC. Her marriage was not a happy one and ended in divorce after the birth of two sons. She had a brief period of institutionalization for mental problems and died in the mid-fifties after several years of poor health.

Little Marjorie, "Marty," died at the age of eight following some type of abdominal operation.

Mildred, the only other surviving member of this generation of this large, talented, intelligent and musical family, graduated from WSC in three and a half years in home economics and nutrition. She continued her education at the University of Iowa where she earned a Master's degree and met her husband, Edward P. Coleman. He had a degree in mathematics from the University of Mississippi and was also working for a Master's degree. Mildred worked in therapeutic diatetics while her husband was continuing his education. During World War Two they were stationed at the United States Military Academy at West Point where Edward taught. After the war he went on to get his PhD in engineering at Columbia University. They moved to Los Angeles in 1951 where he was Professor of Engineering at the University of California at Los Angeles until his retirement in 1979. They have two daughters and two grandchildren.

John, "Bud," was a husky, handsome high school student of seventeen when he died. There is a story that he and some other boys went to a football game in Seattle. On the way back they hopped a ride on a freight train. "Bud" unfortunately found his way into a refrigerator car and subsequently contracted meningitis, survived for a few months, and then expired from pneumonia.

Thomas, "Tommy," attended Washington State College and the University of Oregon and later earned his M.D. degree at Marquette University Medical School in Milwaukee. He also interned there and later carried on general practice in a number of different locations. His wife, Emily, is a registered nurse. In 1973 he was in Alabama and having serious cardiac problems. He returned to Milwaukee where he underwent open heart surgery. He expired in 1979 in Napa, California. Even Tommy seems to have had some affinity for music, for his sister-in-law recalls that the first time she saw him as a small child "He was in his Doctor Dentons pacing up and down the piano keys. No one seemed to object or encourage him, but on he went, up and down the keys." His widow is continuing her nursing career and taking additional academic work of an administrative nature.

The last of this generation of the Robinson family was little Betty Lou. She died at age two and a half of an acute intestinal infection.

As has been mentioned, Bill was the next to the oldest of the children of Lesco and Pamelia Robinson. He, too, was an excellent musician. His principle instrument was the clarinet, but he also played the saxophone

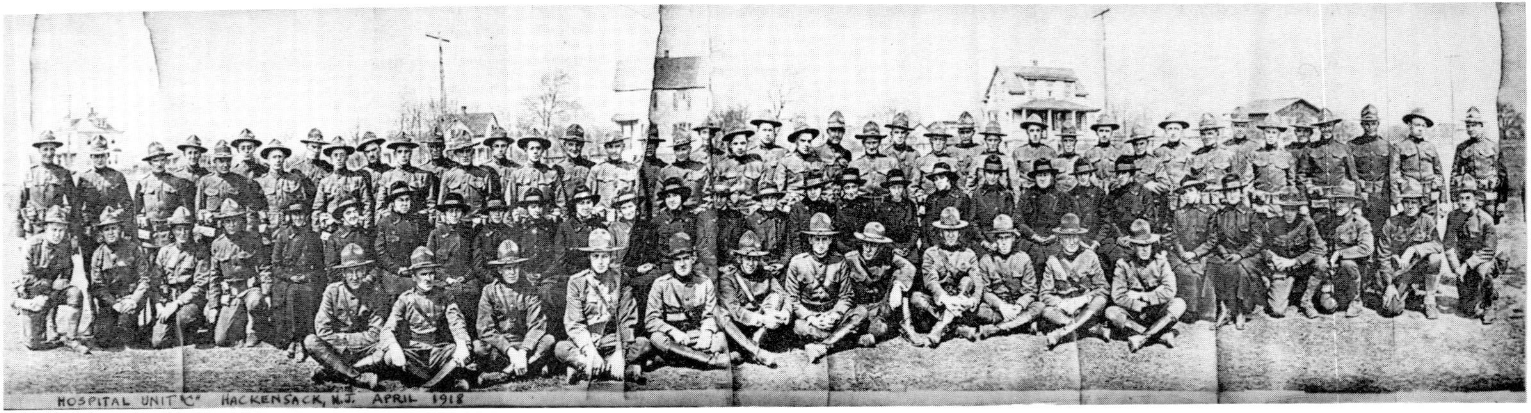

Fig. 4. Faded and damaged photograph of Officers, Nurses and enlisted men of Camp Hospital Unit C just before sailing for France—1918.

and later the piano and organ. He composed an operetta, several orchestral pieces and a stirring march which was played at his graduation from North Central High School. He also composed a duet for flute and clarinet which he and Bonnie performed. At high school he was a good scholar and played football, baseball and golf. He also found time to date an attractive girl named Betty Anderson who was attending Lewis and Clark High School. After graduating from high school Bill attended Whitworth College for one semester and then transferred to Washington State College.

Bill dropped out of college to enlist in the Army for service in World War One. He was assigned to Camp Hospital Unit "C" of the U.S. Army Medical Reserve Corps. (Fig. 4) This unit was recruited almost exclusively in Spokane. Its commanding officer was Colonel Samuel E. Lambert, a prominent Spokane physician who happened to be a good friend of General John J. Pershing with whom he had served in the Phillipines and in the campaign against Pancho Villa on the Mexican border. The unit was made up of twelve doctors, three clerks, twenty-one nurses and fifty orderlies. Among the officers were such well known Spokane physicians as Major Fred P. Sproul, Major Ralph Hendricks, Major William J. Pennock, Captain Fred J. Whittaker, Captain R.N. Hamblen, Lieutenant Arthur Betts, and Lieutenant Edward Barnett. Lieutenant Guy Hollister, who later founded the internationally known Hollister-Stier Laboratories, had come from the Rockefeller Institute in New York to head up the medical laboratory. Private William W. Robinson (Fig. 5) was assigned to this laboratory.

The unit left Spokane December 23, 1917, and underwent training at Fort Riley, Kansas and in Atlanta, Georgia. On April 11, 1918, the unit sailed from Hoboken, New Jersey, on the *S.S. New York* for Liverpool and then from South Hampton to Le Havre whence they were transported in "forty and eight" box cars to Paris. They finally joined the American Expeditionary Forces, of which General Pershing was now commander-in-chief, on April 26, 1918. The unit took over an abandoned chateau which had once belonged to Marie Antoinette and was soon caring for wounded soldiers from the front lines who were brought in "in waves of ambulances," and then sending them on to base hospitals in the rear. Much of Private Robinson's time was spent working in the morgue and assisting at autopsies. Perhaps it was there that he contracted diptheria which was so prevalent among the troops. He was given anti-toxin by Dr.

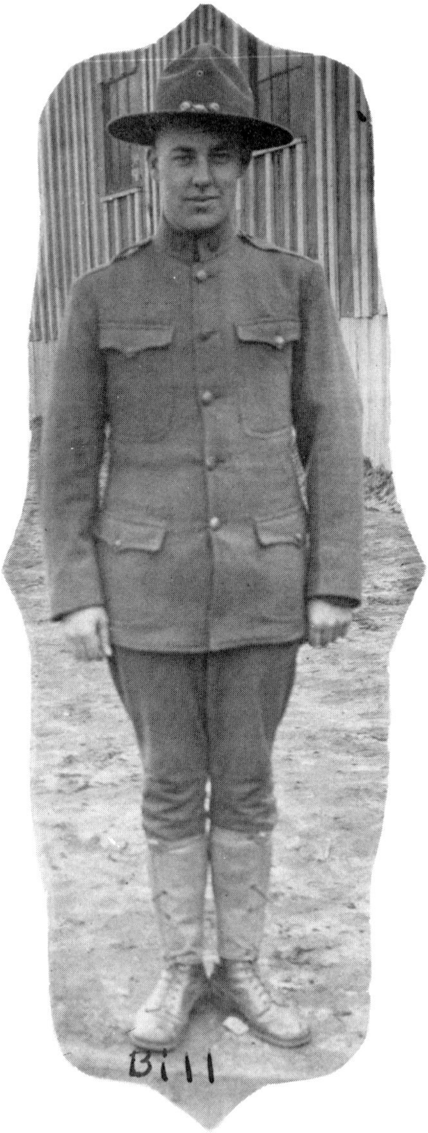

Fig. 5. Private W.W. Robinson, World War One

Hendricks, in spite of which he developed the dread complications of diptheritic myocarditis and neuritis. He was in bed for approximately four months and then evacuated to the U.S. in a hospital ship. He was discharged from the service with a fifty percent total disability rating for which he was to receive compensation for the rest of his life and financial help in paying his way through medical school.

After his release from the military Bill returned to Spokane in 1919 where he married his high school sweetheart, Elizabeth Anderson. Betty was an attractive, popular, highly intelligent young woman. As a wife she was warm, affectionate and industrious. She was aware that because of her husband's poor health prospects (he had been told that he probably would not be able to work past his fortieth birthday) the ultimate burden of supporting him and any children they might have could well fall upon her. When Bill went back to Rush Medical College, she accompanied him and enrolled in the graduate school of the University of Chicago in the Social Service Department. They both worked very hard. Bill maintained a high grade point average and was elected to the honorary scholastic medical fraternity Alpha Omega Alpha. He graduated in 1923. Betty was one of two graduates from her program to be chosen by Jane Addams to work with her at Hull House. Added money was brought in by Bill doing anatomical drawings and medical art work and playing his clarinet which also got him into football games. Betty typed notebooks for other medical students and helped Bill with his home research projects some of which involved the use of guinea pigs which she had to look after.

After earning his M.D. degree Bill interned at Cook County Hospital and then had a two year surgical residency at the Presbyterian Hospital in Chicago. After completing his training young Doctor Robinson obtained a license to practice medicine and surgery in the state of Washington and returned with his wife to Spokane where he opened an office in the Empire State Building in 1926. Like most of his colleagues of that era he was engaged in general practice but his principle field of interest was in surgery. For a brief period Dr. Lesco Robinson joined his son in practice but that didn't work out very well. Bill's modern ideas of medical practice and furious work pace did not coincide with his father's so the older Robinson returned to his old office adjacent to his home. Young Dr. Robinson rapidly acquired a widespread reputation as a skilled surgeon and developed a large practice. Initially most of his patients requiring hospitalization were admitted to the Deaconess Hospital and a contemporary newspaper account credits him with having carried out four hundred operations during the first eighteen months he was on the staff. He also enjoyed privileges at Saint Luke's and at Sacred Heart Hospitals.

Bill was smart, aggressive and hard working. He had a resourceful and inquisitive mind. He invented a number of instruments such as a surgical sewing machine, a ureteral stone extracting basket and a self retaining wound retractor. He also suggested innovations for the radiologic equipment which he had in his office, looking ahead to such developments as cinefluorography. He had a happy marriage, was an expert golfer, bridge player and musician. It truly seemed as though he had everything going his way. But there can be no doubt that his early success aroused a certain amount of envy and jealousy among his fellow physicians.

Bill and Betty Robinson had two children. Their daughter, Betty, was born September 21, 1923, while they were living in Chicago. After she grew up she was happily married and now lives in Southern California. Her husband was the son of a doctor and became a successful business man. He passed away in 1974. They had five children; four sons and a daughter. Her oldest son, not surprisingly, is a talented musician and is also working as an orthopedic assistant. The Robinson's son, Billy, was born in Spokane, January 6, 1928. His mother tells that when he was about fourteen he enlisted in the Marines but when the recruiting officers visited his mother to verify his age the truth came out and he was rejected. Later during World War Two he was accepted into the Navy where he served in the submarine division. After the war he took premedical work at the University of Southern California. There were problems getting into medical school so for a few years he participated in research work. He did not find this field of endeavor sufficiently fulfilling so he entered a seminary to prepare himself for the ministry. He is now a working priest who is devoting most of his efforts collaborating with the police department trying to help young people with drug problems. He is married and has two sons and one daughter and now a grandchild.

2

A CAR ROLLS OVER

ON A COLD, DARK, RAINY NIGHT in November of 1927 an event occurred which had a profound effect on the lives of a number of people and on the relationships within the local medical community. A group of young people was returning home from a social gathering in the Spokane Valley. As they drove along the poorly illuminated Apple Way the bulk of an unlighted parked vehicle suddenly loomed out of the darkness into the glare of their headlights. The driver swerved manfully to bypass this unexpected obstacle. By his efforts a collision was avoided but as his car skidded around its wheels passed over the shoulder of the road and the car overturned. Amazingly, only one of his passengers was seriously injured, a pretty seventeen year old, dark eyed, brunette high school student by the name of Elsie Prather. Pinned under the car she sustained fractures of the mid shaft of the right femur and of the upper end of the right fibula along with multiple grimy and dirt filled lacerations and abrasions of the right leg. At this time none of the hospitals in Spokane had emergency departments as we know them now so she was taken to the "Emergency Hospital," a euphemism for modest facilities maintained in the Spokane City Hall where her wounds were washed out and sutured by the lay "steward" in attendance and Dr. George A. Downs summoned. he examined her, applied a splint and had her removed to Sacred Heart Hospital, where she was given a hypodermic injection and the leg further immobilized with sand bags. There was no mention in the hospital records of impaired circulation at this time. X-ray pictures were taken and the following morning Dr. Downs, a general practitioner, decided to operate. Assisted by Dr. R.N. Hamblen, whose chief interests were obstetrics and gynecology, he carried out an open reduction of the fractured femur through a lateral incision, applied metal bands to hold the bone fragments in apposition and then put on a plaster cast. Nothing further was done to the wounds on the leg.

From the first things did not go well. Elsie suffered an inordinate amount of pain and ran a septic course. A severe infection of the operative wound developed which required reopening the wound and evacuation of copious amounts of pus. As time went on numerous other abscesses developed throughout the leg and thigh which required incision and drainage and several changes of her cast. Ultimately the metal bands were removed from the femur whereupon the bone ends promptly came apart assuming a position with five inches overlap and forty-five degrees angulation. Her course continued toxic and febrile, she lost weight and became progressively more debilitated although at one point her condition had become sufficiently stable to warrant moving her to her home. Large ulcers developed around her foot and ankle, her toes shrivelled and dried up from gangrene, contractures developed, and the end of one femoral fragment came through the skin of her thigh. In the meanwhile on two occasions, Dr. Mitchel Langworthy, then the community's leading orthopedist, had been called in to see her in consultation, but since her foot still seemed viable when he saw her in December there seemed little else that could be done. However, her condition continued to deteriorate until by April of 1928, according to one observer, she was only about "eighteen percent alive." At about this time Dr. Downs suggested amputating the affected limb but the Prather family, by then thoroughly dissatisfied with Dr. Downs, called in young Dr. Robinson who had been a lifelong friend of Elsie's uncle, Claude N. Prather, and had played baseball with him when they were in high school together. Elsie, an only child, had been raised by her grandmother along with her father's brother and two sisters, to all of whom she was devoted.

On May 22nd, Dr. Downs was dismissed as the attending physician and the family insisted that Dr. Robinson take over Elsie's care. Knowing well the ethics regarding the role of consultants and the position in which this would place him with his already disaffected colleagues Dr. Robinson attempted to disassociate himself from the case completely, but because of the seriousness of the problem and his longstanding friendship he finally agreed to continue in attendance and do what he could to help the unfortunate girl. He admitted Elsie to Deaconess Hospital and requested Dr. Langworthy to see her again. It was now apparent that because of the impaired circulation and the profound sepsis that nothing short of amputation would be of any value. It was no longer a matter of attempting to save her limb but of saving her life. Dr. Langworthy agreed completely but was reluctant to become further involved personally, so on the twenty-sixth of May Dr. Robinson proceeded with a below the knee amputation. Following this Elsie made a good recovery and required no further surgical procedures except revision of the thigh wound and removal of the protruding bone fragment.

Dr. Downs, of course, was outraged by this, as he regarded it, flagrant breach of medical ethics and protested volubly to his colleagues. Then to make matters worse he threatened to sue the Prathers to collect the fee for his services to Elsie. This was the last straw for the Prathers and thereupon they decided to file suit against Dr. Downs for negligence and improper treatment.

On May 13, 1929, the suit came to trial in Superior Court in Spokane, Judge W.A. Huneke presiding. Attorney V.T. Tustin represented the plaintiff and Attorney E.J. Cannon the defendant. The damages sought was $33,400, making this the largest malpractice suit which had ever been tried in Spokane. In spite of this and of the intense concern of the local medical community there was little public interest in the case initially. Inconspicuous little accounts of the proceedings were tucked away in the back pages of the newspapers. These were prohibition days and stories of the seizure of stills, the locking of "Blind Pigs," and the activities of Al Capone and Bugs Moran occupied the front pages. Then there was Charles Lindbergh's wedding and Spokane's own Bing Crosby, who, along with the Rhythm Boys was singing with Paul Whiteman's orchestra, and who had just released his first solo record. The only medical event to hit the front page that week was the disastrous Cleveland Clinic Hospital fire in which 124 persons perished.

The day Dr. Robinson was to testify there were over twenty-five doctors in the court room. They knew where his sympathies, sense of propriety and of duty to his patient lay. He later charged that he had already received threats that if he testified against another physician, he would be driven out of the practice of his profession in Spokane. Even his father had been told that if his son testified in the Downs' case every hospital in town would be closed to him. When he was called to the witness stand he realized he was placing his career in jeopardy but he was not intimidated, for he sincerely believed that the doddering defendant was incompetent, undependable, totally unqualified to manage such a serious medical problem and had in fact ruined Elsie Prather. He proceeded to tell the jury that her injury had been grossly mismanaged, that the treatment of choice would have been manipulation and traction. Dr. Langworthy testified that Dr. Downs' method of treatment had been correct, that nothing else would have "worked." The plaintiff's attorney, Mr. Tustin, insisted that in view of all the contamination which had occurred at the time of the accident, that an open operation which led to infection and its disastrous consequences should never have been performed. John O'Shea said the girl would have lost her leg in ten days if anything different had been done. A.R.T. Cunningham supported Downs' treatment. R.J. Kearns said he had never had any luck with "calipers" and traction. Robinson took the stand again and pointed out that since gangrene had developed that either the cast had been too tight, in which event it should have been split, or the femoral artery blocked in which event it should have been explored. At one point the arguments between Tustin and Cannon became so heated that both attorneys were obliged to apologize to the court. Elsie sat by quietly in the court room with her crutches by her side while all this was going on.

The case went to the jury on the afternoon of May 22nd. The next day the jury returned a verdict in favor of the plaintiff and awarded her $12,500. Cannon's law partner, Frank McKevitt asked the court for a judgement in Downs' favor and that the jury's verdict be set aside. If this was denied a new trial would be sought. The press gave Dr. Robinson chief credit for the way the case had turned out and expressed admiration for the courage displayed by a young man only three years out of medical school (residency) to stand up against the combined testimony of the older men.

The medical "fraternity" of Spokane was in an uproar. Things of an unpleasant nature began to happen to Dr. Robinson. He was shunned by other doctors in the city. There were rumors that he was guilty of performing incompetent, unnecessary and improper operations. Adverse publicity began to hurt his practice. A crushing blow occurred when Deaconess Hospital where he had been doing most of his work closed its doors to him. Later St. Luke's Hospital and then Sacred Heart told him he was not wanted. The insurance carrier then cancelled his malpractice insurance. It looked as though the threats he had received were being effectively carried out. It was time for Dr. Robinson to take pause and consider his options. One was to leave town with his tail between his legs, a beaten young man. The other was to start a hospital of his own, an idea which he had had in the back of his mind for some time. Being a smart, cocky, resourceful individual he chose the latter course.

He had already taken an associate into his office in January of this year. Dr. Robert H. Stewart was a Spokane boy who earned his M.D. degree in 1926 at the University of Oregon Medical School. He interned at the Deaconess Hospital and then took some post graduate work at the New

York Lying-in Hospital before joining Dr. Robinson. Then Dr. Robinson's wife, Betty, began to scout around looking for a lot which would be a suitable site for a hospital. As she tells it, one morning she saw a man putting up a sign on a lot just east of and immediately adjacent to Sacred Heart Hospital saying that the property was to be sold for delinquent taxes. She rushed down town to get her husband and brought him up to look at the lot, then went to see her father, Mr. Fred Anderson, to see if they could raise the money to purchase it. As she says, "We finally made it" and an entire city block was obtained. Shortly thereafter notices appeared in the newspapers that the Rockwood Clinic Hospital was being constructed at East 11 Ninth Avenue. Noel Thompson, who had designed the Deaconess Hospital, was the architect and John Anderson the contractor. Dr. Robinson was quoted as saying that the hospital would be giving a new type of service where a complete examination and necessary medical and surgical services would be available under one roof under the close personal supervision of the physician in charge. "Spokane" he said, "is one of the few large cities in the United States that is without such an institution. The desirability of rendering this type of medical service is shown by the outstanding success of the Mayo Clinic in the middle west, of the Robert Coffey Clinic of Portland and the Virginia Mason Hospital Clinic in Seattle.

"Modern medicine is rapidly becoming an exact science, and the day of guess work diagnosis will soon be a thing of the past. It is only by the aid of modern equipment and the use of a well equipped bacteriological and chemical laboratory and by X-ray study that an accurate diagnosis can be obtained. In the clinic hospital, this type of service can be rendered without the necessity of the patient being referred around from one doctor's office to the next."

In the fall of this same year a new trial was allowed in the Downs-Prather case. There were said to have been errors in the record and Judge Huneke ruled that attorney Tustin had made insinuations while examining witnesses which the evidence did not justify. The retrial opened in Superior Court on November 4, 1929, with Judge E.G. Jeffers of Ephrata presiding. There was a little more public attention than at the previous trial although only Dr. R.A. Hahn's trial for criminal abortion made the front page of the newspapers. The same attorneys as in the previous trial, V.T. Tustin and E.J. Cannon were pitted against each other. The defense had shifted its tactics somewhat, this time maintaining that the fractured femur had resulted in a major arterial injury which required an open reduction for decompression and control of bleeding. In fact the arterial injury was now blamed for most of the subsequent troubles. Of course this was before the days of arterial repair and reconstruction, but even so it was never made clear how successful exposure and ligation of the bleeding vessel could be accomplished through a lateral incision. The defense maintained moreover that the operation per se had nothing to do with the infection which followed since strict aseptic technique had been employed and that only sterile instruments and never a hand had entered the operative wound!

Again Dr. Robinson, who was described by the press as the "star witness," testified that Dr. Downs had used improper methods and that external methods of treatment would have been better, being basically simpler and involving less chance of infection. He conceded that open operation was justifiable under certain conditions but not in this instance. Dr. Downs maintained that his consultants, Drs. Langworthy and Hamblen had advised him to continue what he was doing during the post operative period. Dr. Richard Dillehunt, the Dean of the University of Oregon Medical School testified that an open operation would be justified if conditions were as Dr. Downs now stated they were, since this would make it possible to examine the state of the tissues, bones and blood vessels. Dr. R.N. Hamblen testified he had seen the patient in consultation and then helped with the operation. He described evacuating lots of clots and tying off a bleeding artery which he thought was the profunda femoris. Drs. C.B. Ward, Joseph Aspray and John O'Shea testified for Dr. Downs and the testimony of Dr. Mitchel Langworthy approving Dr. Downs' course of action was read into the record.

Dr. Robinson agreed that an open reduction would be indicated if the leg was as described by the defendant but as Mr. Tustin pointed out there was nothing in the hospital record to indicate the presence of a ruptured artery which could obstruct the circulation. In fact he maintained that the present emphasis on a cut artery was an afterthought on the part of the defense to justify the operation. In one dramatic moment demure, slender Elsie Prather took the stand and bared her amputation stump for the jury.

On the fourteenth of November the case went to the jury, Judge Jeffers refusing a defense plea for a directed verdict in favor of Dr. Downs. The jury required only one half hour to reach a verdict in favor of the plaintiff and increased the damages awarded her to $19,000 and costs.

The defense requested yet another trial on the basis that nothing had been proved by the plaintiff and because the jury had only deliberated for such a short time. This request was denied so there was talk of an appeal to the Supreme Court of the State of Washington but nothing came of it. Elsie Prather ultimately received $7,400. Dr. Downs later alleged that he had but $12 to his name, that he was ill and $3000 in debt and in no position to pay anyone anything and of course in those days no one carried much malpractice insurance.

After all this brave young woman endured it is good to be able to report that she is still alive and has had a happy and productive life. She writes "I think of myself as an ordinary person leading a normal life." After recovering from the effects of her accident she moved to Portland where she finished high school. She has been married but for the past ten years has been a widow. She has had no children of her own but has helped raise a number of other people's children including two of her husband's who had been previously married, and more recently his grandchildren. For twenty-three years she worked as a clerk for the Portland Department of Parks until her retirement four years ago at age sixty-five. She first went to work when her husband began to suffer from poor health. Much of what happened during those dreadful years she has forgotten or never knew but she still feels a great debt of gratitude to Dr. Robinson and an affection for his memory.

It would seem pertinent at this point to explain why Dr. Langworthy's testimony had to be read into the record. Just a little over three weeks before the second trial a disgruntled Department of Labor and Industry patient whom Dr. Langworthy had seen for a disability examination in connection with an injury which had occurred two years earlier, walked into his office and fired six shots at him from a twenty-five caliber automatic pistol mortally wounding Dr. Langworthy, slightly wounding his nurse and then killing himself with a shot through the head. Dr. Langworthy was taken to Sacred Heart Hospital where he was given several blood transfusions and operated upon by Dr. E.S. Jennings who removed the bullet from his abdomen and repaired the perforations in his bowel. Twenty-four hours later, on October 9th, this loved and highly respected thirty-eight year old orthopedist died from his injuries. After his death a memorial to Dr. Langworthy was started in the form of a library and educational fund for the children in the Shrine Hospital for Crippled Children at St. Luke's of which he had served as head. Dr. Robinson's offer of a contribution to the memorial fund was declined. A notice in the November issue of the Spokane County Medical Bulletin contained the following paragraph:

> Nearly all the members of the Spokane County Medical Society have sent in checks and we hope to be able to claim every member with one exception a contributor. The officers of the Society and the Library Committee have decided that a contribution from that one member who has proved unworthy of associating with ethical practitioners will not be accepted."

This was signed "C.S." the then president of the Spokane County Medical Society.

3

PARAGON OR ROGUE?

BECAUSE OF THE QUESTIONS which had arisen regarding Dr. Robinson's judgement and his surgical procedures an investigation had been quietly launched. It later developed that the most specific allegations came from a young physician who had been a boyhood friend of Dr. Robinson's and whom Dr. Robinson had kindly asked to assist him at a number of operations when the new doctor first came to town. Some imcompatibility led to a termination of this arrangement and soon the former assistant was accusing Dr. Robinson of frequently performing sterilization operations on young women and even hinted at abortions. Shortly after the first Downs-Prather trial Dr. George Anderson, with the approval of the Reverend Doctor Robert Warner, the Superintendent of Deaconess Hospital, had taken for the purpose of obtaining a second opinion, seven from among four hundred of Dr. Robinson's hospital records to a Dr. George Swift, an official of the American College of Surgeons who happened to be in Portland at the time. The word was brought back that the Deaconess would be removed from the list of accredited hospitals unless Dr. Robinson was barred. So without any sort of hearing Dr. Robinson was informed that the Deaconess Hospital would not admit any more of his patients.

Dr. Robinson was becoming desperate. In the hope of clearing his reputation, on his own initiative he removed these same seven records from the Deaconess Record Room and took them to Chicago to obtain the opinion of some of his former teachers. He visited the headquarters of the American College of Surgeons where he talked with Dr. Malcolm MacEachern who was in charge of the College's Hospital Accreditation Program. Dr. MacEachern denied that any threat had been made regarding the Deaconess Hospital or anything said about unnecessary or improper surgery by any College official. Robinson showed his records to such men as Dr. Arthur Dean Bevan, professor of Surgery at Rush Medical College, Dr. N. Sprout Haney, chief of Gynecology, Dr. Carey Culbertson, author of the text book "The Female Pelvis" and chief of Gynecology at Cook County Hospital, and to other authorities such as Drs. Edwin Miller, A.E. Kantor and Harry Oberhelman. He was told that no fault could be found with his cases from a medical or legal standpoint. He returned to

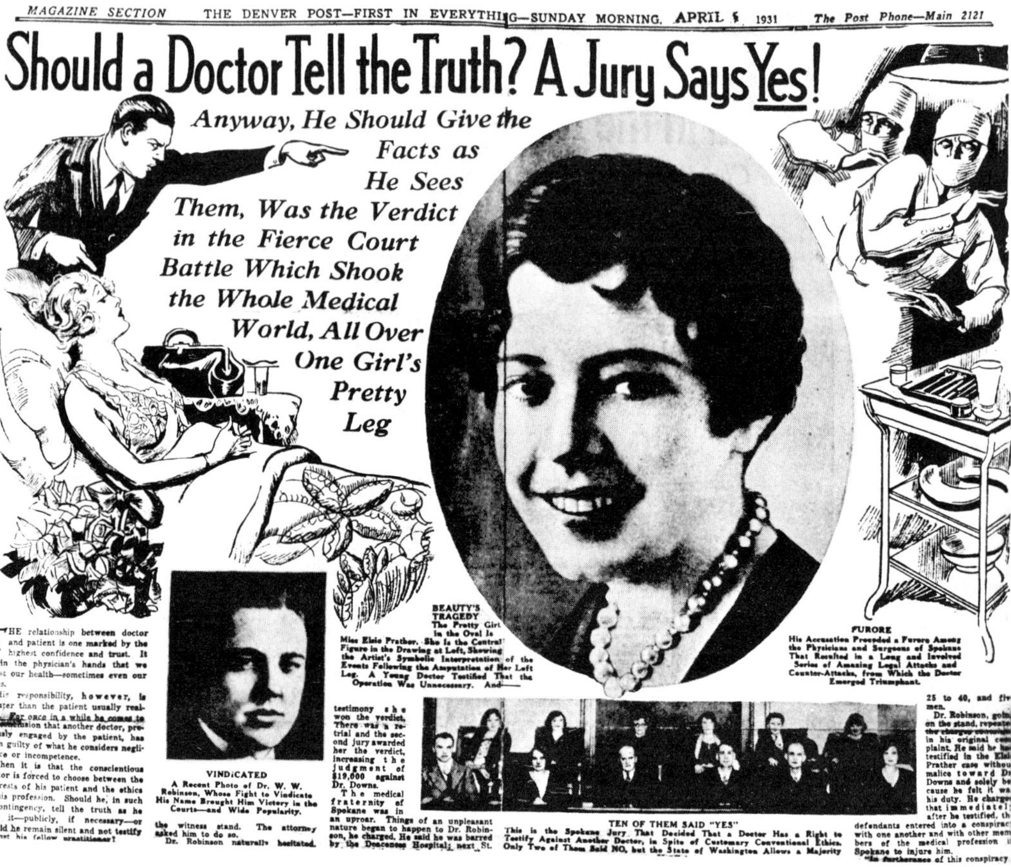

MAGAZINE SECTION THE DENVER POST—FIRST IN EVERYTHING—SUNDAY MORNING, APRIL 5, 1931 The Post Phone—Main 2121

Should a Doctor Tell the Truth? A Jury Says Yes!

Anyway, He Should Give the Facts as He Sees Them, Was the Verdict in the Fierce Court Battle Which Shook the Whole Medical World, All Over One Girl's Pretty Leg

THE relationship between doctor and patient is one marked by the highest confidence and trust. It is in the physician's hands that we trust our health—sometimes even our lives.

His responsibility, however, is greater than the patient usually realizes. For once in a while he comes to the conclusion that another doctor, previously engaged by the patient, has been guilty of what he considers negligence or incompetence.

Then it is that the conscientious doctor is forced to choose between the interests of his patient and the ethics of his profession. Should he, in such a contingency, tell the truth as he sees it—publicly, if necessary—or should he remain silent and not testify against his fellow practitioner?

VINDICATED
A Recent Photo of Dr. W. W. Robinson, Whose Fight to Vindicate His Name Brought Him Victory in the Courts—and Wide Popularity.

the witness stand. The attorney asked him to do so.

Dr. Robinson naturally hesitated.

BEAUTY'S TRAGEDY
The Pretty Girl in the Oval Is Miss Elsie Prather. She Is the Central Figure in the Drawing at Left, Showing the Artist's Symbolic Interpretation of the Events Following the Amputation of Her Left Leg. A Young Doctor Testified That the Operation Was Unnecessary. And——

testimony she won the verdict. There was a retrial and the second jury awarded her the verdict, increasing the judgment of $19,000 against Dr. Downs.

The medical fraternity of Spokane was in an uproar. Things of an unpleasant nature began to happen to Dr. Robinson, he charged. He said he was barred by the Deaconess Hospital; next St.

FURORE
His Accusation Preceded a Furore Among the Physicians and Surgeons of Spokane That Resulted in a Long and Involved Series of Amazing Legal Attacks and Counter-Attacks, from Which the Doctor Emerged Triumphant.

TEN OF THEM SAID "YES"
This is the Spokane Jury That Decided That a Doctor Has a Right to Testify Against Another Doctor, in Spite of Customary Conventional Ethics. Only Two of Them Said NO, but the State of Washington Allows a Majority

25 to 40, and fiv[e] men.

Dr. Robinson, goin[g] on the stand, repeate[d] [illegible] in his original com[-] plaint. He said he ha[d] testified in the Elsi[e] Prather case withou[t] malice toward Dr. Downs and solely be[-] cause he felt it wa[s] his duty. He charge[d] that immediatel[y] after he testified, th[e] defendants entered into a conspirac[y] with one another and with other mem[-] bers of the medical profession i[n] Spokane to injure him.

"In furtherance of this conspiracy

Fig. 6. Part of a page from the Sunday Supplement of the Denver Post April 5, 1931

Spokane reassured and feeling vindicated. Confronted with this evidence the Rev. Dr. Warner then told Dr. Robinson that if he were kept on the staff a number of other doctors had threatened to boycott the Hospital.

The final and most devastating blow fell at a closed meeting of the Spokane County Medical Society in the Old National Bank building auditorium on the night of January 16, 1930. Dr. Robinson was accused of purloining seven records from the Deaconess Record Room and of performing unnecessary and improper operations. The second charge was dropped and in reply to the first charge Dr. Robinson said that he had only taken the records to show them to disinterested authorities in the hope of clearing his name whereas he felt Dr. Anderson had taken them with a view to injuring him. A poll was taken of the ninety-six members present and it was decided to expel him from the Society. He was asked to leave immediately. Dr. Stewart who was also present accompanied him from the room. At the door Dr. Robinson stopped and said, "I thank the thirteen who voted for me." One of those who voted against dismissal said he did so because he couldn't stand the thought of Robinson getting any more publicity.

The following day Dr. Robinson "dropped a legal bomb into the midst of the medical community." He filed suit in Superior Court against ten of Spokane's most prominent doctors charging them with conspiring to injure him and his reputation and making it necessary for him to construct his own private hospital and operate it at a loss since he was barred from the city's other hospitals. He asked for $100,000 damages. The physicians named were Drs. J.H. O'Shea, E.M. Welty, Carrol Smith, S.P. Seaberg, R.N. Hamblen, T.E. Hoxey, E.B. Nelson, G.H. Anderson, T.D. Burger and D.H. Lewis. The resulting trial was one of the most amazing in the history of Spokane jurisprudence up to this time. It produced eleven books of transcripts and 6,660,000 words of testimony. In contrast to the previous trials this one was front page news throughout, with frequent glaring headlines. Coverage was nationwide as well as local and often wildly sensational. (Fig. 6) Four days later the newspapers announced the departure of Dr. Robinson's associate, Dr. Stewart. He was going to Portland for further study and to practice. He was quoted as saying that the present controversy was not the cause of his leaving. He reported that his association with Dr. Robinson had been pleasant and that he was satisfied as to Dr. Robinson's honesty and integrity.

Presently nine more physicians who were County Medical Society or Hospital medical staff officers were named in the complaint, along with the Superintendent of Deaconess Hospital. Included were Drs. C.B. Ward, R.M. Schulte, H.E. Rhodehamel, E.J. Lawrence, F.J. Whittaker, C.A. Veasey, Jr., P.J. Gallagher. Oscar Sternberg, W.J. Pennock and the Rev. Dr. Warner. Representing Dr. Robinson were the attorneys with whom he had worked in the Downs-Prather trials, V.T. Tustin, Clyde Belknap and Winfred Chandler. Representing the defense was the law firm of Cannon, McKevitt, Hamblen and Gilbert.

Things moved slowly at first. There were many delays due to legal arguments and demurers. On March nineteenth, 1930, the suit against the twenty defendants opened in the Superior Court of Judge R.M. Webster. By the following week Judge Webster had approved most of Dr. Robinson's complaints but because of their multiplicity he ruled that separate actions would have to be instituted. In mid April an amended complaint was entered. The claim for damages was reduced to $35,000 for losses incurred from the necessity of building a private hospital and $30,000 for slander. A week later the new suit was filed but again there were postponements due to more demurers. Then in May Judge Webster became ill and the trial was deferred until September. In the meanwhile the judge denied attempts by the defense to have the case thrown out of court. In mid August Dr. Robinson filed another "new" complaint. A month later the attorneys were again clashing in court. The defense now asserted that the reason Dr. Robinson had been kicked out of Deaconess Hospital was that he had pledged not to perform abortions but had violated this pledge, and had in addition, performed thirty or forty sterilizations. They claimed that he had long planned to build his own hospital so as to escape the scrutiny of his peers. Dr. Robinson himself felt that some of Sacred Heart's opposition was due to his "skimming the cream" at his new hospital right next door. Then in October several of the defendant physicians and their attorneys went east to such medical centers as Chicago, Rochester, Minnesota and Baltimore to obtain depositions regarding some of Dr. Robinson's patient records.

Finally by the first of December a jury of seven women and five men had been chosen and the trial began with Judge Dolph Barnett of Yakima presiding. The first few days Dr. Robinson, described by the press as a "dapper young surgeon," spent considerable time on the witness stand before a crowded court room. First he repeated the charges made in the original complaint. He stated that he had testified in the Elsie Prather case without malice toward Dr. Downs and solely because he felt it was his moral obligation. He charged that immediately after he testified, the defendants, who for years had agreed among themselves never to testify against another physician, entered into a conspiracy with one another and with other members of the medical profession in Spokane to injure him by destroying his practice and attempting to "run him out of town." In furtherance of this conspiracy, he charged, "The defendants, believing that if the hospitals of Spokane were closed to the plaintiff, the plaintiff's practice would be injured, caused notice to be served on each of the three hospitals in Spokane, both on their own behalf and on behalf of the other doctors in Spokane, that unless the hospitals refused admittance to the plaintiff and his patients, they would boycott the hospitals." The defending doctors not only denied these charges but sought to prove that Dr. Robinson was guilty of incompetent, unnecessary and improper surgery, citing several specific cases. "OLDER DOCTORS JEALOUS" headlined the Spokane Daily Chronicle.

On the tenth of December Mr. Cannon made yet another of his motions to have the case dropped. The judge denied this but on the following day he cleared St. Luke's and Sacred Heart Hospitals of the ouster charges and dropped from the case Drs. Lewis, Whittaker, Veasy, O'Shea, Gallagher, Pennock, Rhodehamel, and later Drs. Lawrence, Schulte, Burger and the Reverend Warner.

Then the outside experts began to appear. Dr. J. Tate Mason of Seattle testified that most of the plaintiff's operations which he had reviewed were questionable. Dr. W.R. Cubbins of Chicago in a deposition stated that twenty-three cases that he had reviewed were improper. Interestingly enough, his Department head, Dr. Culbertson had supported Dr. Robinson in his deposition as had his colleague, Dr. Oberhelman. Dr. Alfred Strauss of Chicago found little justification for most of the operative cases he had gone over. The most scathing denunciation of Dr. Robinson came from Dr. H.J. Whitacre of Tacoma who found many of the operations "reprehensible, shameful and damnable." The interchanges between the attorneys and between the attorneys and witnesses were spirited and often acrimonious; the histrionics at times unbelievable. As the trial wore on people began to get on each other's nerves. At one point Attorney Hamblen said to Dr. Robinson, who was basically a rather cheerful sort of person, "I wish you would quit smiling at me, Dr.

Robinson." At another, Attorney Cannon pleaded, "I wish the court would admonish counsel [Mr. Tustin] to be a gentleman. I know he can't but tell him to try." The press of course had a hay-day. Dr. Anderson was referred to as "Little Friday" for his role in the original investigation of the Robinson records and when an attractive Deaconess Hospital nurse testified the caption on the news story read, "Woman with Red Hair in Case."

In response to the charges of improper surgery Dr. Robinson said that these charges were fraudulent and originally brought before the Deaconess Hospital Board of Trustees in order to damage him. In rebuttal he paraded a number of his female patients before the court to show that they were happy and satisfied as a result of his treatment. They were presented by number and not by name to preserve their anonymity. This is said to have come as a "bombshell" to the defense which objected strenuously. Dr. Gallagher disparagingly referred to the performance as "Lydia Pinkham testimonials." Cannon in his cross examination of one of the women learned that at one time she had been treated for syphilis and proceeded to castigate Dr. Robinson for allowing her to work as a waitress although Dr. Robinson pointed out that her Wasserman test had been negative at the time.

On December 20th Dr. Robinson is said to have put in some telling blows over the almost constant objections of the defense. No mean actor himself and a competent amateur artist, he spent much of the day instructing the jury in matters medical with the aid of skillfully executed drawings on a blackboard which had been brought into the courtroom for the purpose. There was no question but that he was an effective witness and made a far better impression on the jury than some of his opponents. On December twenty-fourth the court was adjourned for Christmas. In the midst of all the arguments and in-fighting, the sarcasm and bitterness, it seemed almost an irony when Judge Barnett wished the jurors and attorneys a very "Merry Christmas." By this time the trial was being referred to by some of the newspapers as "Judge Barnett's Surgical Clinic."

By the thirty-first of December the trial had gone into its twenty-first day. Further defense motions for dismissal had been denied. Then on New Year's Eve came the startling discovery that one juror was an employee in the kitchen at St. Luke's Hospital. This caused quite a furor but the only action taken was to place the jury under lock and key. Judge Barnett spent over an hour delivering twenty-four instructions to the jury. The jury was directed to consider whether to vote on conspiracy involving all of the defendants, conspiracy involving only some of them or a no conspiracy verdict, at the same time deciding whether to hold the defendants liable for damages because of injury to the plaintiff through slander.

The jury spent New Year's Day of 1931 at the court house listening to the broadcast on the radio of the Rose Bowl Game between Washington State College and the University of Alabama (Alabama won by a score of 24 to 0). The following day the jury was exposed to a heavy barrage of defense arguments. Attorney Cannon pulled all the stops. There were allusions to Florence Nightingale. Mary of the Cross, the Lord's prayer, serving God and preserving souls for the hereafter, religious beliefs and eugenics. Dr. Robinson was accused of excessive pride, self will, arrogance, materialism and finally admonished to "go out into the woods and cut down trees" where he could do but little harm! The headlines announced "ROBINSON CASE BITTERLY FOUGHT: The opposing attorneys stop at nothing in their tongue lashings." Their tongues were described of being at times "coated with vitriol." Throughout the entire trial Betty Robinson had been an almost constant attendant, often dashing off on errands such as obtaining needed reference books.

On January third the jury received the case after twenty-three days in court. The following day the jury arrived at a verdict by a vote of ten to two after fourteen hours and twenty-five minutes of deliberation. On January fifth the Spokesman Review put out an EXTRA to announce the results. $30,000 was awarded to Dr. Robinson for slander and humiliation. Damages for Dr. Robinson's exclusion from the hospitals and the costs of building his own hospital were denied. The ten remaining defendants held involved in the conspiracy and slander charges were Drs. Welty, Smith, Seaberg, Hamblen, Hoxey, Nelson, Anderson, Ward, Schulte and Lawrence. Among other things the jury obviously felt the Downs case had a great deal to do with this one despite the defense protests to the contrary.

Without a doubt Dr. Robinson had won not only a material, but a tremendous moral victory. The press and the public of the city hailed his triumph. Newspapers from distant cities ran full page accounts in their Sunday supplements praising the courageous efforts of the young doctor to vindicate his course of action. Patients showed their support by flocking to his new clinic and hospital many of them leaving their former doctors to do so. As can be imagined however, his stunning victory made him few friends among his colleagues in the medical community. Rifts and animosities were created, vestiges of which persisted for a great many years and which in some instances were not forgotten until most of the principals involved in this painful affair had passed away.

The day after the verdict was rendered Mr. Cannon announced he would seek a new trial or appeal to a higher court. The damages awarded were alleged to be excessive and the jury prejudiced. The juror who was revealed to be an employee at St. Luke's Hospital was alleged to have talked about the case to her fellow workers and to have told them she was going to vote in favor of Dr. Robinson. Moreover the defendants maintained that their alleged actions had nothing to do with Dr. Robinson's testimony in the malpractice suit although the jury believed otherwise. After much discussion, on February 11th Judge Barnett reopened the suit. Because of their complexity he asked for written pleas from the attorneys. On the first of June the verdict was set aside by the trial judge and a new trial granted. Finally on July 29th, 1931, all of the participants agreed to settle the slander suit out of court rather than face the ordeal of another trial. The defendants agreed to pay all expenses of the trial, legal fees, and any expenses incurred by Dr. Robinson in defending himself against the charges which had been levelled against him. The total costs were estimated to be in the vicinity of $50,000. It was said that there would be an assessment of $300 from each member of the County Medical Society. Dr. Robinson received no money although it was later rumored that he had financed his new building with his awards. Actually it was vindication which he sought rather than money and one of the stipulations of the settlement was an agreement to reinstate Dr. Robinson into the Spokane County Medical Society. As a result of these negotiations, on August 13th the court signed an order dismissing the slander case against the ten physicians. It turned out that enough physicians made voluntary financial contributions so that no formal assessment was necessary. Some were said to have paid as much as several thousand dollars. Aside from vindication one reason reinstatement was so important to Dr. Robinson was that at that time it was a prerequisite to hospital staff membership.

In spite of the settlement agreement Dr. Robinson never did get back into the County Medical Society until after World War Two. He applied for membership shortly after the agreement was reached but was told to submit his application at the time of the annual meeting of the Washington State Medical Association. This he did in December of 1931

but was then told that he would have to apply through the County Society. This he promptly did but his reinstatement was denied by the local group. This political shuttling continued, although throughout, his membership in the American Medical Association had never been affected. On one occasion, several years later he attempted to attend a meeting of the County Society but the group went into executive session and denied him admission. Just prior to his entry into military service at the outbreak of World War Two the then president of the Spokane County Medical Society, Dr. J.G. Matthews responded to an inquiring newspaper reporter that Dr. Robinson's most recent application for reinstatement had been rejected at a meeting of the medical society although the Spokane Daily Chronicle of that date referred to Dr. Robinson as "one of the most widely known surgeons in the Inland Empire." Finally upon his return from overseas in World War Two efforts again were made to block his admission to the society. At this time, however, sentiments in the community were strong in favor of returning veterans and when it was pointed out by other veterans that the principal opposition came from a group of physicians who had escaped military service entirely, he was finally admitted to membership in the Spokane County Medical Society. After all this he probably never attended more than one or two meetings of the Society.

Another interesting phenomenon occurred immediately following the notorious law suit. Dr. Robinson, who had enjoyed an excellent record as far as any hospital liability or malpractice litigation was concerned, was suddenly confronted with a spate of nuisance litigation. In April of 1931 a woman who owed a substantial hospital and medical bill threatened suit for $6,150 alleging paralysis of a hand. Papers were served but no suit was definitely filed. In May of that year the woman who had appeared as a witness in the slander suit and from whom the defense had elicited the fact that she once had had syphilis, sought $30,000 in damages for alleged defamation of character. The resulting publicity, she said, caused her to be shamed and to lose her job. This case was thrown out of court by the judge. Then in 1932 a third woman threatened suit when at attempt was made to collect a bill for treatment. Nothing ever came of this action.

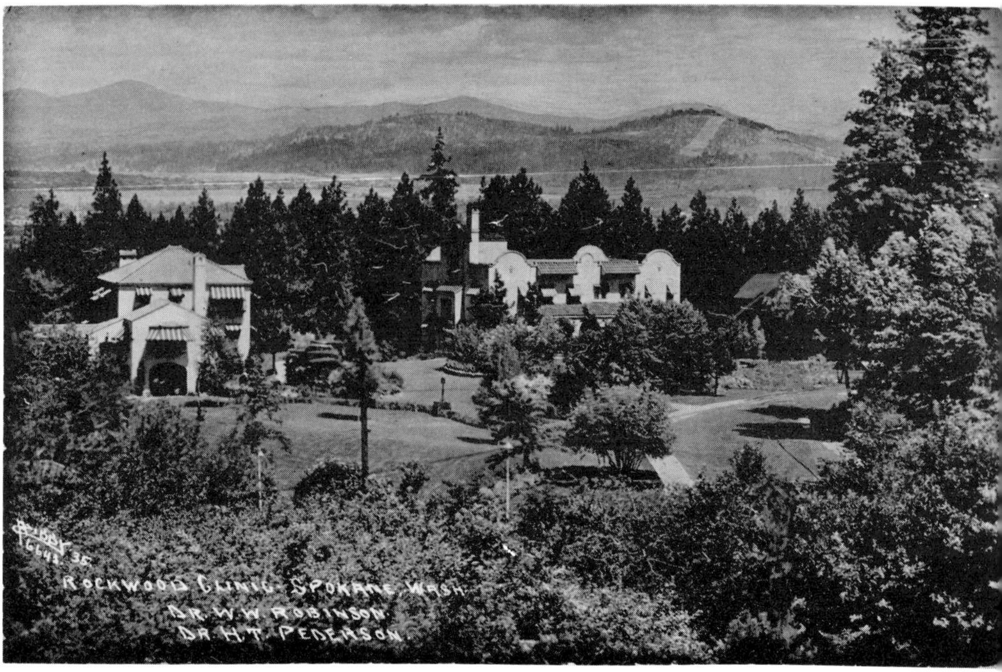

Fig. 7. Robinson Home and Rockwood Clinic Hospital—1935 Mount Spokane in Background.

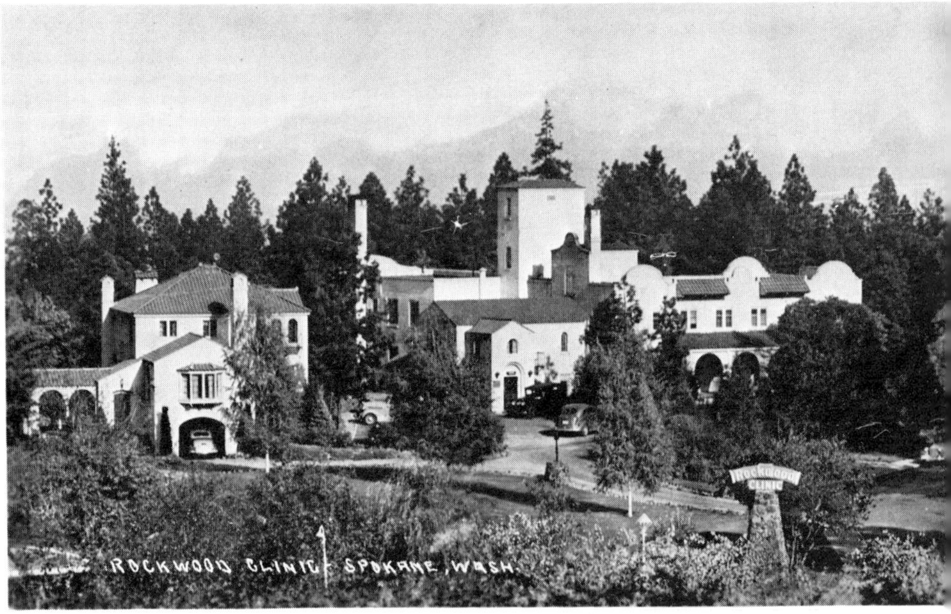

Fig. 8. Later View Showing Addition to Hospital

4

THE BEGINNING OF THE ROCKWOOD CLINIC

THE ROCKWOOD CLINIC HOSPITAL, built at a cost of around $50,000, had opened its doors to ten patients with a staff of four in 1930. It was an attractive Spanish style building of reenforced concrete with a stucco exterior, a red tile roof and arched porticos, doorways and windows. It was three stories high on Ninth Avenue and five stories on Eighth. (Fig. 7) The spacious and well kept grounds were beautifully landscaped. Inside the building was a bright but rather austere lobby with an adjoining business office. There were soon enough comfortable and attractive rooms to accommodate forty patients. There was a well equipped laboratory, modern X-ray equipment, an operating room for major surgery and another for minor procedures, and examining rooms for out patients. Originally Dr. and Mrs. Robinson occupied quarters on the top floor. The building soon had to be enlarged (Fig. 8) at a cost of $25,000 to accommodate ten more beds which could be expanded to a total of seventy-five after the Robinsons moved into the home which they had built immediately to the west of the main building. The grounds were later embellished with a putting green and a handsome swimming pool. A picture taken in the early thirties suggests a millionaire's estate rather than a medical facility. (Fig. 9)

Patients who were cared for in the hospital still recall the cheerful surroundings, tasty food and the good care they received. Rates were $5.00 for a double room, $7.50 for a single with bath. Office calls were $2.00 and house calls $4.00. A complete examination with laboratory work and whatever radiologic studies were necessary seldom exceeded $35.00.

Mrs. Robinson put her whole heart into the project. She did a lot of the planting of trees, shrubs, and flowers on the grounds, purchased the furniture for the hospital and all of the sheets and bedding. She did the shopping for food for a long time, helped out in the kitchen and at each month's end assisted the girls in the business office. She tells that she took care of all the food trays. There were individual flower vases and place cards and tiny toasters and percolators so the patients could have hot coffee and toast. She only recently learned that her two children enjoyed her working on the attractive trays since it gave them a chance to get into the diet kitchen and filch ice cream.

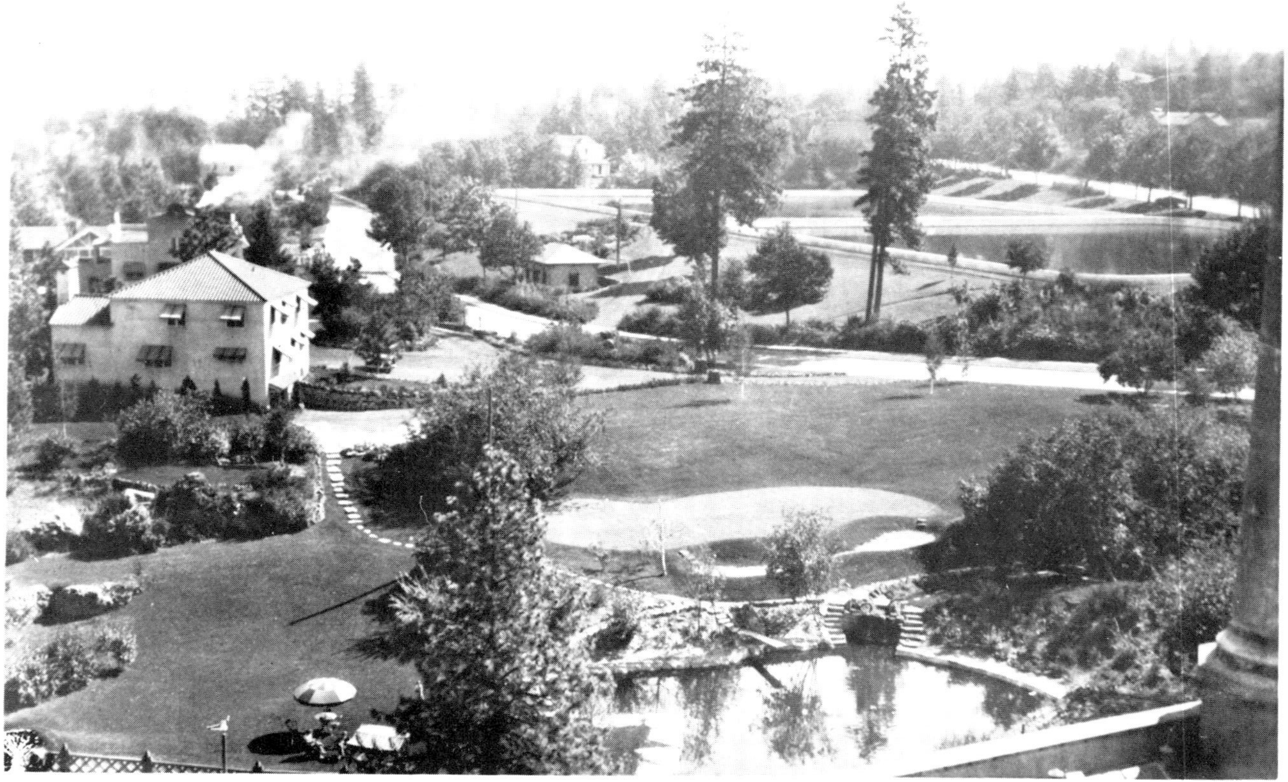

Fig. 9. W.W. Robinson Home on 9th Avenue showing beautiful grounds, swimming pool and putting green. City reservoir in background.

In the midst of all of his other problems, in August of 1931 Dr. Robinson met with a freak accident. One day while working on the X-ray machine in his new clinic, unaware that someone had improperly adjusted the timing device, he received a tremendous jolt of electricity which resulted in a fracture dislocation of his left shoulder. An open reduction was ultimately required and although it resulted in some permanent limitation of function he was able to resume his status as one of the best golfers in the city. But it was this accident more than anything else which made him realize that he needed some help in caring for the ever increasing patient load at the new clinic and hospital. His shoulder was not doing as well as he thought it should so he went back to Chicago for further treatment. While he was there he contacted an old friend from his days at Presbyterian Hospital and invited him to join him in Spokane.

This old friend was Dr. Harold T. Pederson who graduated from Rush Medical College in 1923. After completing his internship he spent two years in general practice in Utah. He later returned to the Presbyterian Hospital for two years additional training and then opened an office in Chicago. It was then that Dr. Robinson encountered him. Dr. Pederson was aware of Dr. Robinson's difficulties with the local medical community but thought highly enough of him to accept his offer and came to Spokane in September of 1931. Knowing what he did, it was with considerable trepidation that he took his state board examinations for licensure. He later said he never studied so hard for any test in his life. Fortunately he passed without difficulty and he was subsequently admitted to membership in the Spokane County Medical Society. It was, however, quite a few years before he was able to gain admission to any social organization such as the Spokane Country Club or the Early Birds Club.

* * * * * *

Rowland Bond, the well known feature writer for the Spokane Daily Chronicle, tells a nice little story about these days. There was an Italian grocer named Nick from whom the Robinsons had been buying most of their groceries. With all of his trouble and the construction of his hospital, Bill was getting a bit strapped for money. He warned Nick that his credit might not be very good. Nick said that he was never worried even when the debt was approaching $5,000. "Better cut me off." Bill is alleged to have said. Nick never did, ultimately was repaid and felt that he was more than rewarded for his charity when later on he would walk into a crowded waiting room at the Rockwood Clinic and whenever Dr. Robinson would spot him he would say, "Nick, you come in."

Mrs. Robinson tells that there were frequent big Indian "pow-wows" in Spokane when they first came and that Bill soon had quite a following of Indian patients. He used to tell of a spectacular incident of which she probably never heard but to the truth of which he attested. It seems that a number of Indians were having a wild party in one of the skid road hotels late one bitter winter night. In spite of the sub-zero weather outside, the temperature in the room continued to rise until most of the revelers chose to divest themselves of their garments. As the party became more loud and raucous the police appeared on the scene to break it up. One enthusiastic participant in the orgy, anxious to avoid incarceration escaped out of a window onto the fire escape. Nude and perspiring he sat down on one of the iron steps and promptly became adherent to the metal. The fire department and Dr. Robinson were summoned. The firemen wrapped the shivering miscreant in blankets but it was not until the resourceful physician arrived and applied hot moist towels from a lower landing that the poor man was thawed loose.

As he grew more prosperous, and could afford it Bill developed a passion for boats and boat racing. His daughter, Betty, tells of one day when the family was on its way to a big race, towing his "pride and joy" on a trailer behind the car at a lively clip. As they were speeding along, suddenly a boat and trailer passed them. It not only sped by them but finally ended up in a clump of brush beside the road. Bill was outraged to think that anyone would be so stupid as not to secure a trailer hitch properly. When the family finally realized that is was Father's "pride and joy" which had gone by everyone had a good laugh since fortunately the boat was undamaged and above all had inflicted no damage on anyone else.

She also tells about her father operating on a friend of his who was an ardent fisherman and had the habit of keeping hooks, lures, lines, etc. in his mouth while he was attaching his bait. When the man had emerged from his anesthetic, Bill brought in a tray full of hooks, lines, lures, etc. and explained that this was what he had had to remove.

Although Bill usually spent his money as fast as he made it and so seldom had much cash worth, he was an astute business man. There was, however, one venture which was a notorious financial flop. Shortly after he opened his hospital he bought a farm with the idea of supplying the hospital with produce, eggs and dairy products at reduced rates. At one point he announced that in his hospital one could drink the best $1.25 a quart milk obtainable, and he soon divested himself of the farm. In the present days of wildly inflated prices there seems little humor in this but when milk was costing ten cents or less a quart it was quite hilarious.

Bill also had a racy story about life in high society. It dealt with an attractive young divorcee who was attending a ball at the Hayden Lake Country Club. As she whirled gaily around to the admiration of all the spectators in the arms of her dancing partner of the moment, a contraceptive diaphragm was suddenly seen to go rolling across the dance floor. Its ownership was never claimed.

* * * * * *

As a result of all of his legal problems Dr. Robinson had taken pains to familiarize himself with laws applying to charitable hospital corporations in the state of Washington and learned that at that time as long as a hospital used reasonable care in the quality of employees it hired and the services it provided it was virtually impossible to sustain a legal action against it. In fact, one Hugh D. Combs, vice president of the United States Fidelity and Guaranty Company, in charge of claims, stated in an address reported in the Company "Bulletin," "A hospital is immune from liability by reason of the negligence of its doctors and nurses with respect to any matter relating to patients' medical care and attention." This was indeed a far cry from the vulnerability of hospitals and their governing bodies in the legal climate of the 1970's. Dr. Robinson became so interested in this aspect of things that in September, 1934, he enrolled in Gonzaga University Law School which he attended until February, 1936, at which time he withdrew before graduating. He later became a charter member of the American Board of Legal Medicine.

On the twenty-fifth of March, 1932, an Agreement of Association of a charitable corporation called the Rockwood Clinic was drawn up. Its purposes were to receive and care for the sick and wounded, to employ duly licensed physicians to furnish such medical and surgical treatments as patients might require, to buy, build, own, lease or mortgage such real or personal property as might be required in the conduct of said business, to employ such nurses and other assistants as might be required to carry out its purposes, to borrow money and receive donations for its support; to devote all its income and profits after paying the expenses to the purposes of such institution....50,000 shares of capital stock without normal or par value were to be issued. The first meeting of the subscribers was held on the 2nd of April and the agreement signed by William W. Robinson, M.D., President, Fred W. Anderson (Mrs. Robinson's father) Vice President and Mrs. Elizabeth C. Robinson, temporary Secretary and Treasurer. Trustees, not less than three or more than twenty-three were to be elected by the stockholders at the annual meeting to be held in May of each year. A few days later a certificate of approval was issued by the Secretary of the State of Washington. In July it was stipulated in the bylaws that any profits were to be used in the expansion and improvement of the Clinic's present facilities and the development of an experimental laboratory for research in medicine and surgery. Five percent of the beds were to be reserved for charity cases.

At the beginning of 1933, the assets of the Clinic were $77,648, liabilities $57,799, net assets $19,649. Dr. Robinson offered to buy 49,500 shares of stock for $19,649 to be paid for by his turning over to the Rockwood Clinic the Clinic Building, adjacent grounds, his dwelling house and all equipment owned by him and used by the hospital, his Cadillac sedan and Ford Cabriolet. The trustees agreed to consummate the purchase, assume all current liabilities and issued him 49,500 shares of stock.

By 1935 the Rockwood Clinic enjoyed an excellent reputation in the community at large. Accompanying an application for hospital liability and malpractice insurance was a letter from Mr. Tod Oien of the McGovern and Carroll Insurance Company, who for many years handled insurance matters for the Clinic, in which he states, "We cannot recommend this risk too highly. The moral and business hazzard [*sic*] is 100%." Of particular concern to potential insurers had been the question of whether Dr. Robinson, in the event of his being sued for malpractice, would be able to obtain sufficient testimony from reputable doctors in Spokane. Mr. J.E. McGovern had previously investigated this contingency and after talking to a number of doctors who were not involved in Dr. Robinson's previous litigation concluded that he thought Dr. Robinson would have no difficulty in securing medical testimony in his favor in case an unjustified malpractice suit was brought. Subsequent events proved

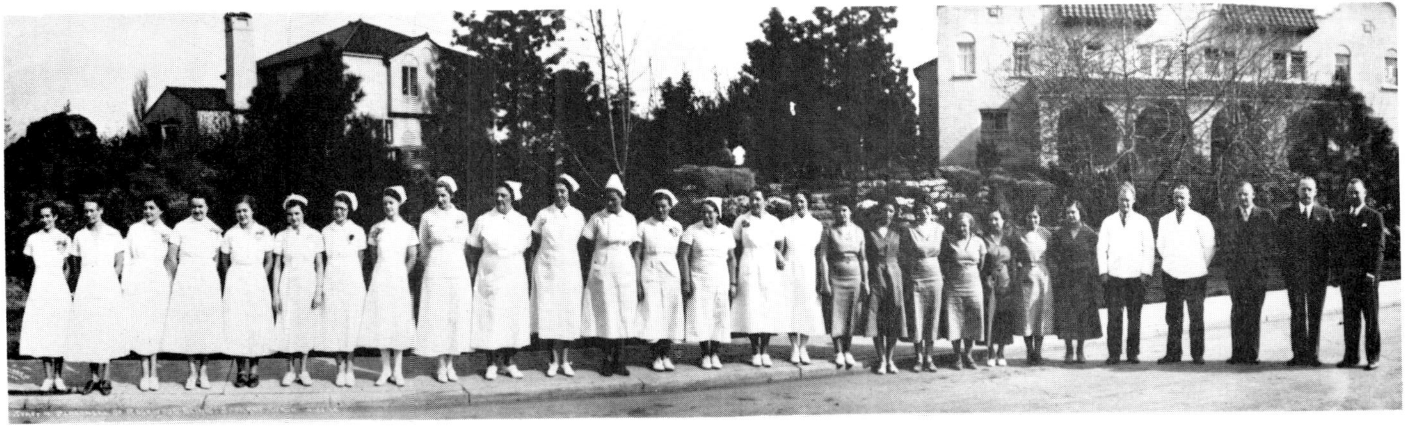

Fig. 10 Rockwood Clinic Staff—1935

him to have been correct in his estimate of the situation.

In January of this year Dr. Robinson's father, Lesco A. Robinson, died from influenza and a heart ailment at the age of 63. His wife, Pamelia, had passed away in 1923 and he had then married a Lenore Harney, who was still living at the time of Dr. William Robinson's death in 1957.

A panoramic photograph of the Rockwood Clinic staff taken in 1935 shows, among others, Dr. Robinson, Dr. Pederson and Mr. Earl G. Ogsbury who had signed on in 1932 as superintendent of the Hospital and business manager of the Clinic. (Fig. 10) He had previously managed the Montgomery-Ward store and also maintained an interest in some Buster Brown Shoe Stores in Washington and Oregon. Perched on a ledge behind the group are two little boys who probably were not supposed to be in the picture. One is Dr. Robinson's son, Billy, and the other is Dr. Pederson's son, Harold. Harold's mother had died before the move to Spokane and in 1933 Dr. Pederson had married one of the Clinic nurses, Miss Bertha Frank, the wedding being held in the Robinson home which appears in the left background, the hospital being the building on the right. Standing third from the left is a beautiful young brunette, Miss Mabel Lennon from Farmington, Washington, who was working at the Clinic as a receptionist and stenographer. (Fig. 11) The group shot hardly does justice to this comely female. Her manners and her disposition matched her good looks and it was not very long before Dr. Robinson had fallen desperately in love with her.

In January of 1936 the stock holders met to fill a vacancy created by the death of Mrs. Robinson's father, Fred Anderson. Mr. Ogsbury was the one elected. At their next meeting a week or so later salaries were established. Dr. Robinson as president of the trustees and head physician was to receive $1200 a month and Dr. Pederson as assistant physician, $600 a month. It was also decided that all profits would be placed in a reserve account earmarked for building and equipment maintenance and that a similar account should be set up for deferred income. The following year Clyde Belknap, a member of the legal team which had represented Dr. Robinson in his law suit, was elected Trustee and Vice President. Mr. Ogsbury was elected Secretary and Mrs. Robinson, Treasurer.

Dr. Robinson's attraction to Mabel Lennon continued to grow in intensity. At first they could only meet surreptitiously which was neither to

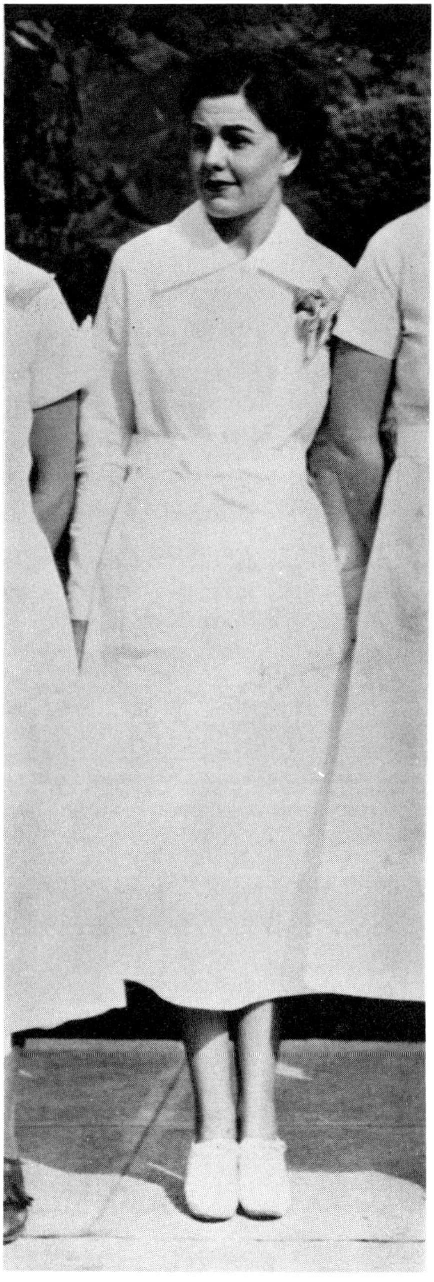

Fig. 11. Enlargement of third figure from left in Fig. 10, Mabel Lennon

her taste nor his. But before long things had reached a point where he decided to seek a divorce from his wife, Betty. This was accomplished in 1938 and shortly thereafter he married Mabel. Interestingly enough this action of dumping Betty and marrying Mabel earned Dr. Robinson more enmity and criticism from the community at large than anything which had happened before. The effect on Betty was devastating. She was totally devoted to him, had stood by him through all of his troubles, worked beside him during his early struggles and later projects and borne him two children. A dedicated and emotionally stable woman, she was inconsolable and is said even to have considered taking her own life. With the support of her multitude of friends she gradually began to pick up the pieces of her life. First she moved to San Francisco taking the children with her. When she had found housing Dr. Pederson brought down her car and her two dogs. Later she moved to Santa Monica. She had a number of friends in other Southern California communities but preferred not to be near them feeling they would feel obligated to do things for her and the last thing this courageous woman wanted was sympathy or pity. It is good to be able to report that she is still living and happy in Santa Monica. She remarried, at this time to a Los Angeles high school principal, Cecil Phayre Lyon and though now legally blind derives great happiness from her two children, her eight grandchildren and her one great grandchild.

Dr. Robinson adored his new wife and the marriage seems to have been a happy one. Mabel's role was not an easy one. Dr. Robinson provided for her well but with his long-standing ostracism by the medical profession and subsequent disapprobation by many former friends, their social life was at times beset with complexity. However, with Dr. Robinson's widely acknowledged high professional standing in the eyes of the public, with the life style he was able to maintain, with his outgoing personality and his manifold other talents, combined with Mabel's reserved, decorous and refined nature they gradually regained a wide circle of loyal friends.

5

GROWTH AND PROBLEMS WITH THE I.R.S.

MEANWHILE THE CLINIC AND THE HOSPITAL were prospering. Early in 1937 a general practitioner named Vernon A. Coverstone was added to the staff. He had graduated from the University of Oregon Medical School in 1934 and he was to practice general medicine and obstetrics. A few months later Roy C. Biehn, a 1936 graduate of the University of Wisconsin Medical School, joined the group to offer further coverage in medicine and also in radiology. Dr. Pederson by this time had become a one third partner but all subsequent additions to the staff came as salaried physicians. Dr. Pederson was doing some obstetrics, a little surgery, mainly assisting Dr. Robinson, but his chief interest was in gastroenterology. Dr. Robinson did practically all of the surgery and in addition a good bit of urology and gynecology. The new men had no difficulty in obtaining their licensure to practice medicine or in gaining admission to the Spokane County Medical Society but their reception by the medical community is reported to have been cool. This was not as upsetting as it might have been since because of the rather isolated nature of their practice which was confined to the Rockwood Clinic and its Hospital, none of these men had much day to day contact with the other doctors in town.

In the late summer of 1939 serious questions arose regarding the tax status of the Rockwood Clinic. A special meeting of the trustees was held which was also attended by M. Warner Onstine, the accountant for the Clinic and Attorney Elmer E. Johnston, subsequently a member of the Washington State Legislature, who had been asked to look into the matter. To everyone's dismay, Mr. Johnston announced that the Clinic had been operating in an illegal manner. Under the laws of the state of Washington a corporation could not practice a profession or employ professional people, pay them a salary for their professional skill and collect for itself fees earned by them. Mr. Onstine had met with the Deputy Collector of the United States Department of Internal Revenue who said that the Rockwood Clinic, Inc. was not entitled to any charitable exemption and would be obliged to file corporate income tax, Social Security and Capital Stock tax returns retro-active to January, 1937. Onstine and Johnston were directed to file the necessary returns along with an appropriate protest to the Deputy Collector and to determine, by court proceedings if necessary, the true charitable status of the hospital and its rights as a tax payer.

Three weeks later another special meeting of the trustees was held at which Mr. Johnston recommended:

> 1. The practice of the doctors carried on as part of the Clinic business would have to be discontinued. Separate sets of records were to be kept for the doctors and for services rendered by the Clinic. The activities of the doctors and of the Clinic were to be completely separated.
> 2. The salaries of Drs. Robinson and Pederson were to be terminated.
> 3. A complete change in the financial organization of the institution was to be effected.

The trustees resolved to put these recommendations into effect immediately, to make appropriate adjustments in the Clinic books back to 1937 and as a result of these adjustments to acknowledge a debt to Drs. Robinson and Pederson of $42,717. The doctors stated that they had a partnership between themselves and would henceforth maintain their own books. An agreement between the Rockwood Clinic and the doctors was approved whereby:

> 1. The Clinic would furnish Dr. Robinson and his associates the buildings, equipment and necessary supplies for Dr. Robinson's "family table."
> 2. Dr. Robinson was to act as superintendent of the hospital without monetary recompence.
> 3. Drs. Robinson and Pederson were to guarantee the payment of $10,000 a year for office space and any additional sum necessary to prevent any deficit in the operation of the hospital.
> 4. Dr. Robinson personally was to pay his assistants.
> 5. Drs. Robinson and Pederson were to furnish without charge care to any charity patients in the hospital.

The following month the trustees adopted proposed amendments to the Agreement of Association, Articles of Incorporation and By-laws drawn up by Elmer Johnston so as to qualify the Rockwood Clinic, Inc. as a tax exempt organization. It was stipulated that the shares of capital stock should serve for voting purposes only and should not represent any pecuniary value to the holders thereof. All proceeds were to be devoted to the charitable purposes of the organization and not to the financial benefit of anyone connected therewith. In the event of liquidation or dissolution any properties or chattels remaining after the payment of debts should be applied to charitable use and not go to the stockholders. At this meeting Clyde Belknap resigned as a trustee "In order," he said, "to give Dr. Robinson a free hand in handling the problems now confronting the institution." M.W. Onstine, Elmer E. Johnston and Dr. Pederson were elected as new trustees. A Declaration of Trust was signed and included in the minutes in which the signers disclaimed any right of private property in and to the shares of stock of the corporation and indicated their desire to carry out the purpose of the hospital as indicated in the original Articles of Association. It was another year before the Clinic received notification from the state tax commission that it was not subject to any business or occupational tax and that it was exempt from paying either the state or federal unemployment compensation tax, and finally the long hoped for information from the Commissioner of Internal Revenue in the United States Treasury Department that after reconsideration the corporation was deemed exempt from Federal Income Tax and that contributions thereto were deductible by donors.

This same year an internist named John A. Mills was added to the staff. He was a 1933 graduate of the University of Chicago Medical School and had spent some time at the Mayo Clinic. He is said to have been a very thorough and methodical individual who would sometimes spend all day working up two or three patients. He also had a propensity for periodic brief but mysterious disappearances. At about this same time John E. Anderson, the contractor who had built the hospital and Dr. Robinson's home was added to the Board of Trustees. Dr. Robinson now was willing to accept the house in which he lived and the land on which it stood adjoining the Hospital for $23,000 representing cancellation of the amount due him from the Hospital Corporation, a maneuver which Mr. Onstine said was consistent with the separation of the personal interests of the physicians from those of the institution. The trustees accordingly voted to convey a deed to the property to Dr. Robinson subject to the mortgage rights of John E. Anderson. The next year, 1941, Arlene White, a secretary at the Clinic replaced Mrs. Elizabeth Robinson on the Board of Trustees. In June Dr. Francis M. Lyle, a Chicago trained surgeon with considerable experience in orthopaedics, came aboard. Tom, as he was called, had graduated from Rush Medical College in 1937 and during his residency at the Presbyterian Hospital had worked with Dr. Oberhelman who had familiarized him with Dr. Robinson's old troubles with the Medical Society. The opportunity offered in Spokane, however, seemed too attractive to turn down. Dr. Lyle found his work at the Rockwood Clinic professionally rewarding but the ostracism by the medical community seems to have bothered him more than it did some of the others. The final addition to the staff arrived later that same year, a general practitioner named Albert H. Seering, who graduated from the University of Minnesota Medical School in 1934.

In spite of their professional isolation and the suspicion and animosity with which they were regarded the group of doctors working at the Rockwood Clinic worked well together and felt they were practicing good medicine. Along with their families they formed a close knit and harmonious social group and formed friendships which among the survivors have remained firm up to the present. Morale was particularly high among the nurses and other employees who felt they were part of an elite organization and took considerable pride in the Rockwood Clinic. Many still entertain proud recollections of the quality of the work, the congenial atmosphere and the parts they played.

6

WORLD WAR TWO WIPES OUT THE "OLD" CLINIC

SUDDENLY DAWNED THE "DAY OF INFAMY," December 7th, 1941, when the Japanese bombed Pearl Harbor and Americans realized they were truly embroiled in the great struggle against the Axis powers. Everyone's life, future and well laid plans became uncertain, but for a while business went on as usual at the Rockwood Clinic. A picture of the staff taken in 1942 shows all of the doctors except Dr. Coverstone who had been called into the Army by this time. It also shows the expansion which had taken place in the number of employees. There were now seventy people on the payroll compared to the four when the Clinic opened.

There was even involvement in further litigation. A twenty-eight year old housewife and her husband, Helen and James Hood, brought suit for $27,500 against the Rockwood Clinic and Drs. Robinson, Pederson and Coverstone. The case was heard before a jury in the Superior Court of Judge R.M. Webster during March of 1942. The allegation was that the plaintiff's condition was wrongly diagnosed and that later a sterilization operation was carried out without the knowledge or consent of the patient or her husband. The doctors' findings which were thought to indicate a normal pregnancy in a young woman anxious to have children proved to be due to a hydatidiform mole for which Dr. Robinson operated on her. Justice Raymond F. Kelly was counsel for the plaintiffs while a brilliant defense was carried out by, of all people, Frank J. McKevitt of the law firm Cannon, McKevitt and Frazier, supported by Attorneys Tustin and Chandler. The case dragged on in court for fifteen days. Dr. Richard D. Reekie was the principle expert witness for the plaintiffs. The most telling support for the defense came in the testimony of Dr. Frank R. Fursey. Dr. David H. Lewis also appeared on the stand for the defense. At one point Mr. McKevitt made a motion for non-suit but after lengthy legal arguments this was denied by the judge, but as the trial wore on he did dismiss from the case Dr. Coverstone who had attended the patient originally. Dr. Coverstone had by this time been inducted into the Army and was stationed at Fort Lewis, Washington, from which post he obtained leave and appeared at the trial in his captain's uniform. Dr. Robinson is reported to have made a stellar performance before a crowded court room, explaining the complexities of the patient's problem to the jury and illustrating his testimony with colored pictures which he "rapidly and skillfully" drew on large sheets of paper. Mr. McKevitt actually made it look as though the testimony of the plaintiff's own medical expert indicated that the treatment provided by the defendants was proper. Mrs. Hood even testified as to her confidence in the Rockwood Clinic where she previously had had her tonsils and appendix removed. Dr. Coverstone, she said, had been "very nice" to her.

When the trial finally drew to a close the jury was unable to arrive at a verdict and was discharged. Negligence on the part of the doctors had been stricken from the suit by Judge Webster so the principle issue which the jury had to decide was the matter of sterilization without consent and this it was unable to do. "We'll go to trial on the remaining issue next month," said Justice Kelly but nothing of the sort ever happened. Dr. Pederson's experiences in this suit had a good deal to do with his decision thereafter to limit his practice strictly to internal medicine.

New problems of an entirely different nature now began to confront the Rockwood Clinic. Up to this point the progress of the institution had been marked by growth, success and expansion. Now due to the exigencies of World War Two and the resulting staff attrition it became increasingly difficult to carry on with the work load. One by one the members of the medical staff were inducted into the military service or as it was euphemistically expressed in those days, "joined the colors." Coverstone had already gone and in rapid succession Mills and Lyle followed him into the Army and Biehn went into the Navy. Seering was ill with some type of renal disorder so was not vulnerable to the draft. On October 5th Dr. Robinson reported to the Trustees that a critical situation confronted the Clinic due to war conditions. The hospital was operating at a loss and in debt. Practically all of his medical help had been taken and he felt that he would probably be called into service. He recommended that the institution should be leased or sold to prevent a total loss. The Trustees voted to approve this course of action. By November 1942 no one was left but Drs. Robinson and Pederson and then Dr. Robinson received orders to report to Barnes General Hospital, Vancouver, Washington, for Army duty on November 12th.

A special meeting of the stockholders and Board of Trustees was held November 7th. Ex officio members Mayor F.G. Sutherlin and Chairman of the County Board of Commissioners, Wylie Brown did not attend but approved in writing of the actions taken. Dr. Robinson reported that the adjoining property owners, the Sisters of Charity of Providence, had offered $63,000 for the Rockwood Clinic Hospital which would pay off the first mortgage and all pending debts if he would sell all of his own personal property as well in order to give the Sisters title to all the frontage involved. Dr. Robinson agreed to this and for another $63,000 turned over his home and premises which were also heavily mortgaged. Dr. Pederson favored these transfers rather than suffer a complete loss even though it would cause him personally to lose considerable money that he would need to set up a new practice. The Trustees voted unanimously to authorize the sale of the Rockwood Clinic Hospital building and premises and all of its furnishings and fixtures to the Sisters. They also ratified the former sale of the residence property of the corporation to Dr. Robinson in consideration of the cancellation of the $23,000 debt by him. Mr. Ogsbury was to continue at his salary of $325 a month to supervise the closing of the hospital and to collect the accounts receivable on a 30% commission basis. He was to establish a down town office to carry out these duties and maintain the Clinic records. All moneys left after collection expenses and funds from the sale of equipment were to be invested in War Bonds until the Trustees decided whether to:

1. Reopen as a Hospital and Clinic after the end of the war.
2. Donate the bonds to a similar charity institution.
3. Donate the bonds to charity for the advancement of medical science.

In any event the hospital portion being "charitable" was untouchable except as above. X-ray equipment, personal surgical instruments and office equipment were to be stored.

A month later the sale to the Sisters was still being discussed. It was discovered that there had been an error in the description of the property so a new deed had to be drawn up. A joint announcement by Sacred Heart Hospital and the Rockwood Clinic Hospital had appeared in the local newspapers as follows:

> Due to the heavy calls on the staff of the Rockwood Clinic Hospital by the United States Army and Navy, the Board of Trustees deem it no longer advisable to continue the maintenance of the Rockwood Clinic Hospital.
>
> Effective November 15, 1942, the Rockwood Clinic Hospital will cease operating as a Hospital and at a later date the Hospital and facilities will be added to those of Sacred Heart Hospital.
>
> The Clinic facilities will remain open in their present location until December 31, 1942.

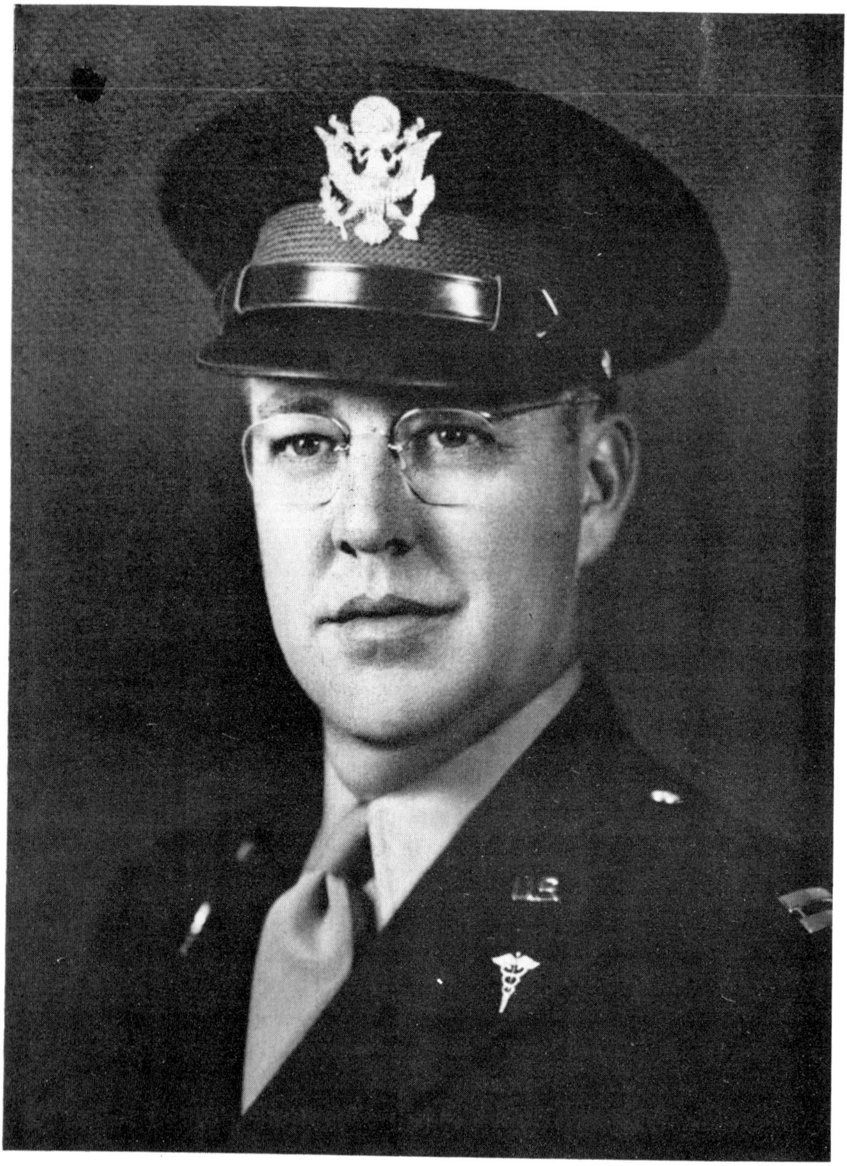

Fig. 12 Capt. William W. Robinson
World War Two

Final official approval of the sale of the Rockwood Clinic and of the Ogsbury contract was obtained at the annual meeting of the stockholders May 11, 1943.

In the meantime Dr. Robinson informed the newspapers that he was requesting deferment because he felt a responsibility to the Clinic and its many patients. How someone who was drawing a monthly check for disability incurred in the First World War would seem a suitable candidate for a captain's commission and active duty in the present conflict is a little mystifying. The Spokane Chamber of Commerce was becoming increasingly concerned by what it called "The continuing raid on Spokane's medical fraternity by the Army and Navy." Chamber President Frank S. McWilliams sent strong telegrams of protest to the Manpower Commission and to Washington Senator Mon C. Walgren pointing out that Spokane had already contributed 160% of its assessed quota of doctors to the armed services and implied that the care of the civilian population was being jeopardized. A response from Senator Walgren's office stated that doctors were not being drafted unless they were declared unessential to civilian practice by the County Medical Board. The Spokane Daily Chronicle commented, "Whether Dr. Robinson's case was passed on by the County Medical Board was not a matter of public record." In any event his request for deferment was not granted.

Sister Superior Henrietta of Sacred Heart announced that the premises purchased from the Rockwood Clinic would initially be used as sleeping quarters for the overflow of student nurses who currently were being housed in several rented buildings. The furnishings were to be transferred to Sacred Heart Hospital to augment its present equipment and the remaining additional space would facilitate the accommodation of a larger number of patients. The lonely task of winding down the operations of the Rockwood Clinic was carried out by Dr. Pederson and Mr. Ogsbury. On the eve of his departure for military service, Dr. Robinson, (Fig. 12) a perennial optimist, stated. "After the conclusion of the war, it [the Rockwood Clinic] will be reorganized and the clinic type of practice resumed in a new and suitable location. All of the doctors who are now in the armed forces have planned to return to Spokane. Dr. Harold T. Pederson will maintain his present office space in the Clinic until January 1. He then plans to establish himself at some suitable location in downtown Spokane."

These events, so important in the lives of those concerned fall into insignificance when one catches glimpses on the backs of the newspaper clippings announcing them of some of the other things which were taking place at that time. Berlin Radio was denouncing as nonsense accounts of the rout of the German and Italian tank army in North Africa. The British Eighth Army, it said, had been obliged to desist from any large scale initiative because of the defensive moves of Field Marshal Erwin Rommel. The United States Navy announced heavy bomb hits on several large Japanese aircraft carriers in the South Pacific and the possible sinking of seven other enemy ships. A report from the North Atlantic described the torpedoing of an Allied merchant vessel. Several of the officers barely escaped in a lifeboat from the sinking ship. The German submarine then surfaced near them, took the ship's captain aboard as a prisoner and then rammed and demolished the life boat. It is sometimes hard to remember the excitement and anxiety of those stirring days.

The experiences of the Rockwood Clinic medical staff while in military service are not relevant to the present narrative. However, a letter to his former associates written by Major Robinson from the hospital in which he had been serving in the European Theater of Operations is of sufficient importance in setting the stage for what transpired after the war to justify reproducing it in its entirety.

302ND STATION HOSPITAL
APO 510, U.S. ARMY

15 April 1944

Dear Pete, Tom, John, Roy, Cover, and Tommie:

I guess that I have been hitting the ball a little too hard and as a result I have landed in the hospital with a coronary and you know what that means. Several good cardiologists have told me that I should retire from active practice and it looks as if I am going to receive a C.D.D.

There is only one job that I would like to see finished and that is the re-establishment of the Rockwood Clinic. I feel that there is a real future for an organized group in Spokane and I feel that it is my duty to see that you boys have a place to come home to where your security will be assured. I am proud of each and every one of you and feel that after this war is over there will be just two classes of physicians; first, those who did their duty in the military service; and second, those who stayed home and lived off the "fat of the land."

Unless you are different from most of the Army medical officers, you will find in the post-war period that most of you will be more or less "broke." There is a considerable fund of money and equipment that belongs to the Rockwood Clinic. This should tide you over in the post-war period. If you want to come back to the Clinic there will be a place waiting for you.

WORKING TOGETHER

I have been fortunate in making the acquaintance and friendship of Major Wendell S. Sharpe who is a graduate of Johns Hopkins, certified by the American Board of Surgery, and who is on the staff of the Mayo Clinic. Major Sharpe is one of the best men they have at Rochester and Dr. Balfour of the Mayo Foundation is anxious to have him back. Although he is sold on the idea of group practice, he does not like the idea of living in the town of Rochester and he is going to take my place in the reorganization of the Clinic. I have seen him work enough and have observed the way he handles men and patients to know that he will make my ideal successor. He has plenty on the ball! He is thoroughly familiar with the medical-political situation in Spokane and, like the rest of you, he doesn't give a "God-damn" just as long as he knows that we are on the up-and-up. I am sure that you will all like him. He will be head and shoulders above anyone in Spokane at the present time as far as surgical ability is concerned. I see no reason why, with your combined efforts, you can't make the Rockwood Clinic the outstanding medical centre of the Pacific Northwest. As for myself, I intend to retire and fade out of the picture but, if health permits, I will do all within my power to add whatever prestige I have with the general public of Spokane in seeing that you get a proper start. I propose to build a new modern clinic in the neighborhood of the Sacred Heart Hospital, adequate for an eight-man group, allowing space for future expansion should you ever decide to rebuild a new modern hospital of your own. The tentative plan I have in mind, should you be interested is: Pete;—General Surgery and Medicine, should he desire again to do group practice; Coverstone:—Obstetrics and Gynecology; John Mills;—Head of the Section of Medicine; Roy Biehn;—X-Ray; Tom Lyle;—Orthopedics and General Surgery; Wendell S. Sharpe, Chief of General Surgery; Tommie Robinson;—Eye, Ear, Nose and Throat.

To those of you who have been out of your field due to war conditions I promise you that I will loan you the money to send you to some post-graduate school to pick up in your professional work where you left off.

With me out of the picture none of you need to feel that you are a "medical outsider;" Although I warn you that with the set-up you will have you will be the cause of jealousy and envy of the medical profession there. It has to be that way—if you don't amount to a damn no one pays any attention to you but when you start stepping on their toes professionally, and particularly financially, then from there on you are a S.O.B. I know because I went through it.

If this does not appeal to you and you do not want to join with the group again please let me know immediately because at the present time in the Service there are good men, at a dime a dozen, eager for such a chance. This will be my last letter to you along these lines but inasmuch as I expect to receive a C.D.D. soon (or kick the bucket) I must know for my future plans. I will guarantee you one year's salary at the same figure as when you left the Clinic and if the Clinic is successful, a pro-rate bonus at the end of the year.

Good luck to all of you and hoping that we can all get together again and make the Rockwood Clinic the Mayo's of the Pacific Northwest.

I thank all of you for your past loyalty.

Sincerely yours,
Bill
Major W.W. Robinson MD

P.S. I am sending this same letter to Pete, Tom, John, Roy, Cover and Tommie. Please don't tell Mabel about that portion of this letter referring to the coronary. She thinks it is my old condition that the Army has just now discovered.

Bill.

Now it is an interesting thing that Dr. Robinson's dream regarding the re-establishment of the Rockwood Clinic as an organized group "with a real future in Spokane" was ultimately realized, but with an entirely different cast of characters than he had envisioned. Of the six doctors to whom his letter was addressed not a single one chose to accept his offer. "Pete," Harold Pederson, was by this time well embarked on a distinguished career as an internist in Spokane and later became the outstanding director of the Medical Service Bureau. "Tom," F.M. Lyle elected to set up what developed into a successful solo practice of surgery in Spokane. John Mills became chief of medicine at the Veterans Hospital in Portland and not long thereafter expired. Roy Biehn returned to Spokane in the private practice of internal medicine. "Cover," Vernon Coverstone, went East for some sort of graduate work and then practiced in Oregon. He was killed in an automobile accident in the 1950's. "Tommie," Thomas Robinson was Dr. Robinson's younger brother. He had not previously been a member of the group but even he chose not to sign up. He ultimately ended up in general practice in Alabama. He underwent open heart and carotid artery surgery in 1973 and died a few years later. Al Seering seems not to have been included in the blanket invitation to return. He had only worked at the Clinic for a few months before the group disbanded and was not in good health. He later was employed as an Emergency Room physician at the newly opened Holy Family Hospital on Spokane's North side and worked there until his death in 1968. Earl Ogsbury, the former business manager, moved to the Tucson, Arizona area where he was involved in a number of highly successful business ventures. He later returned to Spokane for the resection of an abdominal aortic aneurysm and died suddenly a few days after leaving the hospital.

When the present survivors of the old group were interrogated as to why none of them had nibbled at what seemed like the attractive bait offered by Dr. Robinson the concensus seemed to be "We just didn't trust him." Nobody ever accused Dr. Robinson of being dishonest or guilty of peculation, but nobody ever really knew just what he was going to do next. He ran what was essentially a one man show. He was brilliant, capable and energetic, but not above stretching a point if he felt it was in a worthwhile cause. The only derogatory descriptions of him from his former associates were that he was a "real wheeler-dealer" and completely unpredictable. Also the idea of a totally unknown individual being proposed as their new boss and "outranking" all of them must have been a little less than palatable.

They all felt that Dr. Robinson was a good doctor and an able surgeon. In fact one of the things which got him in trouble with the doctors outside of the Clinic was the fact that he was often the first to try and espouse new operative procedures and therapeutic concepts which others either had not heard of or regarded as radical, unproven and unacceptable. For example he was doing gastric resections for peptic ulcer when gastroenterostomy was still the popular procedure locally. But there was a fine line between being ahead of one's times and possibly stretching the indications for an operation. Dr. Robinson enjoyed a high style of living and always seemed to feel that there was a lot more money in the Clinic coffers than there actually was. Even his allusions to Major Sharpe who was associated with him in the 302nd Station Hospital, a young man whose qualities at times truly approached genius, were not without some degree of hyperbole and inaccuracy. Although Dr. Robinson probably believed sincerely as he wrote, "As for myself, I intend to retire and fade out of the picture," no one who knew him well could imagine him totally divorcing himself from the management of the Clinic affairs whether he saw any patients or not.

Dr. Robinson was correct in assuming that his prestige with the general public would be an important factor in the re-establishment of the Clinic. He still had a great many friends in the community and a backlog of loyal patients who were looking forward to his return. Where he thought he was going to get the money to "build a new modern Clinic in the neighborhood of Sacred Heart Hospital" must also have raised doubts in the minds of his former associates since the amount available from the sale of the Hospital and the collection of accounts receivable was far less than had been anticipated. Furthermore the use of the Hospital portion of these funds was closely restricted by the old Articles of Incorporation and tax laws. As of December 31, 1944, there was $23,680 invested in United States Government bonds.

By the twentieth of February, 1945, Dr. Robinson had returned to Spokane and was being discharged from the Army Medical Corps. A special meeting of the trustees was held at the temporary Clinic office in the Paulsen Building which Mr. Ogbury had established. Present were Dr. Robinson, Mr. Onstine, Mr. Anderson, Mr. Johnston, Mr. Ogsbury and Ms. White. Dr. Pederson also attended although he had already announced his resignation from the Board a few days earlier due to the pressures of his own work. Dr. Robinson announced his desire to re-establish the Clinic and a committee, consisting of Robinson, Ogsbury and Anderson was appointed to seek a site. Dr. Pederson's resignation was accepted and Mr. Roy Brown elected to take his place.

May 7, 1945, brought the glorious news of the end of the war in the European Theater of Operations and plans were being put into operation for the invasion of Japan.

7

ROCKWOOD REBORN

ON MAY TWENTY-FOURTH the search committee reported to the Trustees the acquisition of the residential property across the street from Sacred Heart Hospital at West 66 Eighth Avenue. The residence on the premises was a handsome three story building on a bluff overlooking the city. It had been built in 1912 for an attorney named Robert Nuzum. Later it became the home of Edward F. Burns an early Spokane railroad contractor who helped build the Great Northern and The Canadian Pacific Railroads. After his death his widow operated the "Jewel Box," an exclusive gift shop in the Davenport Hotel. Her daughter, Mrs. Irene Burns Miller was at one time one of the few female City Editors in the newspaper world and later went into social work. As a result of her experiences in this field she recently published a spicy book about slum clearance in Seattle.* In recent correspondence she tells about taking her mother as a patient to the old family home after the Clinic had taken it over. "Does it make you feel sad, Mother?" she asked with a lump in her throat. "Of course not!" her mother replied "Each time I come here I say a prayer of thanks that this lovely old house is owned by my doctors for their clinic which is doing so much good."

It was estimated that it would cost $40,000 to buy and renovate the building as a clinic. The war bonds were sold, $20,000 secured by a mortgage on the property borrowed from the First National Bank and the sale was consumated in the name of the Rockwood Clinic, Inc. Dr. Robinson purchased the furniture which was in the home along with the equipment in storage in the Paulsen Building for $2,943. The Trustees then agreed to rent the structure to Dr. Robinson for $400 a month until he had acquired a staff to resume operations. At this same meeting Mr. Ogsbury resigned from the Board due to the demands of his new business ventures. Ms. Arlene White also resigned since she had only been acting in Dr. Robinson's absence. Pauline Kirkpatrick, an office manager in the old clinic and a notary public was elected a Trustee and Secretary-Treasurer of the Board. On August first the lease was signed and Dr. and Mrs. Robinson moved into the newly purchased home. Their living quarters were on the main floor and Dr. Robinson opened his medical office in the old ball room on the floor below.

★ Profanity Hill. The Working Press, Everett, WA. 1979

September 2, 1945, was V.J. Day. After two of their cities had been devastated by a hitherto unknown weapon, the atomic bomb, the Japanese surrendered unconditionally. Although it is still difficult to realize the magnitude and the horror of the forces which were unleashed, at least it was hoped that a lasting peace would be ensured and that people could begin picking up the pieces of their lives.

Although none of the prewar doctors were induced to return, Dr. Robinson had little difficulty in recruiting a cadre from the personnel of the 302nd Station Hospital to help him get the show on the road. There was Dr. James Martin, an internist, Dr. John Remington, a general practitioner, Mr. Donald MacEachern, a former medical corps sergeant who served as a general factotum, and three nurses, Miss Anderson, Miss Kosky and Miss Thomas. Later others were added, some of whom had worked in the old Clinic. There was Charles Tilson who ran the X-ray department, John Canwell who ran the laboratory and Miss Elma Turner, the chief stenographer. Miss Jean Heath, a St. Luke's Hospital School of Nursing graduate, was taken on as head nurse. Mr. John Hay was hired as business manager and Mrs. Dixie Reeves as bookkeeper. Mrs. Jackson and Mrs. Soderquist served as receptionists. Dr. Benjamin Wood, a board certified pediatrician was added to the professional staff. As these acquisitions took place they gradually occupied the rest of the building. In the meanwhile Dr. Robinson had purchased the residence immediately to the east of the Clinic building on West Eighth Avenue where he and Mrs. Robinson made their home from then on.

In March of 1946 Dr. Wendell S. Sharpe, to whom Dr. Robinson had alluded in his letter of 15 April, 1944, to his former associates, arrived in Spokane. Dr. Sharpe was a native of Michigan and graduated from Hillsdale College in that state. He attended Johns Hopkins Medical School, earning his M.D. Degree in 1935. While there he was elected to Alpha Omega Alpha and Phi Beta Kappa honorary societies. He interned in surgery at Johns Hopkins Hospital and then spent a year at Henry Ford Hospital in Detroit. In October, 1937, he went to Rochester, Minnesota where he had obtained a fellowship in general surgery at the Mayo Clinic. In 1941 he served as first assistant to Dr. Howard Gray and then served briefly as an assistant staff surgeon before entering the Army in 1942. While in Rochester he married his charming wife, Mary Lou Wold. Dr. Sharpe was brilliant, able and proud, an outstanding scholar, a born leader, an organizer, an astute business man and an accomplished surgeon with excellent judgement and manual dexterity. He had engaging manners and a warm, compassionate approach to patients which rapidly brought him a devoted following.

On March 22, 1946, a special meeting of the stockholders of the Rockwood Clinic Foundation was held. Dr. Robinson wished to change the name of the corporation to the William W. Robinson Foundation, saying that he wanted the project identified with his name insofar as possible. He also felt that it would be prudent to disassociate more completely the non-profit Foundation from the profit-making Rockwood Clinic Partnership. The motion to effect this was unanimously carried, Anderson, Johnston, Onstine, Ogsbury, Pauline Kirkpatrick being in attendance in addition to the chairman, Dr. Robinson. Appropriate amendments to the Agreement of Association and the Articles of Incorporation were filed and approved by the Secretary of State of Washington State. At the annual meeting of the trustees and stockholders in May Dr. Robinson reported that he had been paying $400 a month rent to the Foundation, improving the property and inviting other Drs. to practice with him. Proceeds of the rental payments were to be put to some charitable use. Improvements to the property were to be limited to $20,000 for which the Foundation would be liable, anything exceeding this amount would have to be paid by the tenants. Ms. Kirkpatrick retired as Secretary and Mr. Onstine took her place.

The Trustees of the Foundation next met in August at which time the lease to Dr. Robinson, "operating under the style of the Rockwood Clinic" was renewed. It was agreed that $41,000 was due to Dr. Robinson for the improvements he had made, this to be paid at the rate of $100 a month at 2% interest. Dr. Wendell S. Sharpe, who by this time had joined Dr. Robinson as a partner, was elected a Trustee. John Anderson resigned as Vice President and Dr. Sharpe was chosen to replace him.

The next doctor to be "invited" was Carl P. Schlicke. Born in Brooklyn, New York, he and his mother moved to California when he was fifteen years old after the death of his father who had been struck down by an automobile. He graduated from Los Angeles High School, and then received an A.B. degree from the University of California at Los Angeles in 1931. In the fall of that year he travelled by boat through the Panama Canal to Baltimore to attend Johns Hopkins Medical School. On the way he met a lissome, blue eyed blond from Redlands by the name of Hilda Hinckley whom, after a whirlwind courtship of six years to the day, he married. While attending Hopkins he and Sharpe became close friends. For three years they roomed together and earned their keep as steward and house manager respectively at the Alpha Kappa Kappa medical fraternity house. After graduation Schlicke also obtained a surgical internship at Johns Hopkins Hospital and the two of them roomed together in the Halsted Surgical Building. Schlicke then spent a year as an assistant resident in surgery at the Long Island College Hospital in Brooklyn, New York. In the fall of 1937 Schlicke also started a fellowship in surgery at the Mayo Clinic. In 1941 he served for a year as first assistant to Dr. Charles W. Mayo. Then for a few months before entering the Army in 1942 he served as an assistant staff surgeon.

During their years together Sharpe and Schlicke had often talked of practicing together. While Sharpe went to Europe, Schlicke served at Fort Riley until the Mayo Clinic Unit was mobilized and when that occurred in 1943 he accompanied the unit to New Guinea and the Philippines. The two friends kept up a correspondence while they were overseas and when Sharpe came to Spokane he invited Schlicke up to look the situation over. This he did that spring, liked what he saw and decided to give it a try. Early in June when his terminal leave from the Army had expired he went back to Rochester for a little intellectual and professional updating. While there and visiting with old friends on the staff he heard some disquieting things about the situation in Spokane. Dr. Jay Bargen having urged him to look up his old friend, Dr. George Anderson in Spokane, which he assured him would be a delightful town in which to practice, then volunteered "There's just one person I hope you're not going in with; a fellow by the name of Robinson." Schlicke assured him that he was aware of the problems Dr. Robinson had had but that was now all water under the bridge.

On the fifteenth of June, 1946, the Schlickes with their three year old son followed a snow plow through Glacier National Park and arrived in Spokane that evening. There was no problem about the state boards except the bore of having to take them. Membership in the County Medical Society was a bit slow in coming and the welcome at its meetings hardly overwhelming. The first painful rebuff came at the meeting of the Washington State Medical Association which was held in Spokane that September. Dr. George Anderson was the President and after one of the sessions Schlicke introduced himself to Dr. Anderson and brought greetings from Dr. Bargen. Dr. Anderson was most cordial until in response to his question, "Where do you have your office, doctor?" Schlicke replied, "At the Rockwood Clinic." on which Dr. Anderson turned on his heel and walked off. Amazingly, the two became good friends in later years.

That summer and fall there were a lot of feelers out for additional internists. Sometimes two would arrive on the same weekend to survey the local scene and the staff's resources would be stretched thin trying to entertain them and keep them apart. One fine day a dapper young man in his Air Corps summer uniform arrived. This was Major Joseph H. Delaney, who was attached to the Air Safety Command. He had attended Montana State University and Harvard Medical School. His father had been a doctor in Bozeman. Joe was a Board certified internist who had trained at Henry Ford Hospital. As a bachelor he had been a bon vivant, was fun to be around and loved to tell his little jokes. He was persuaded to join the group, reported for work in December and soon became the fourth partner. This time he brought with him his new bride, nee Eleanor Welch.

In the meanwhile a special meeting of the Trustees had been held in October at which Dr. Schlicke had been introduced as the new member of the partnership. The resignation of Mr. Ogsbury from the board was formally accepted at this time and Dr. Schlicke elected in his place. The resignation of Elmer Johnston was also accepted.

As the changing of the guard was gradually taking place the members of the original post-war cadre gradually slipped away. John Hay, the business manager, who spent most of his time with his feet up on his desk was the first to leave and Mr. MacEachern assumed his duties. Ben Wood, the pediatrician, left as soon as his year was up. At that time most of the doctors pitched in to get the patients seen regardless of their specialty, sorting them out later on the basis of their complaints. Ben would not participate in such activity and since in the absence of an obstetrician there were very few children as patients he had very little to do. Jim Martin took some additional training in respiratory physiology and went to work at the Firlands Tuberculosis Sanitarium over on the coast. John Remington moved to Davenport, Washington, continuing in general practice, later going to work as an emergency room physician at Holy Family Hospital. Miss Thomas left and was married. Miss Kosky perished shortly after leaving the Clinic from suffocation due to a cigarette ignited mattress fire. Miss Anderson stayed on for several years before leaving and getting married.

Since Dr. Robinson was at that time doing all of his hospital work at St. Luke's the rest of the staff physicians followed suit, although they had privileges at Sacred Heart and Deaconess as well and occasionally admitted patients there. On one occasion Dr. Sharpe was asked by a nurse to see one of the older doctors' patients at Sacred Heart because of some critical emergency which he fortunately was able to resolve. The only thanks he received was an admonition from the doctor never to go near one of his patients again.

There were other episodes which had a rather devastating effect on the ego of a proud man like Sharpe. Schlicke will never forget the first County Medical Society Meeting they attended together. The atmosphere of hostility and disdain was almost physically palpable. As they walked out after the meeting Sharpe commented, "Don't let it worry you, we'll be running this outfit before very long." Sharpe never saw this time come to pass. Then there was a truly tragic and devastating occurrence. Sharpe was asked to see the daughter of one of the town's leading doctors, presumably at the insistence of her husband who was an intern at Sacred Heart Hospital. He felt she probably had a flareup of regional enteritis which required an operation. He asked Schlicke to assist him and as the operation commenced Sharpe remarked, "When they want the best they know where to go!" Within twenty-four hours the young woman was dead. Some of the nurses at Sacred Heart still remember the total emotional breakdown of this usually undemonstrative man after he left the bedside of his deceased patient. And finally there was the gnawing realization that the total control of the Clinic was never quite in his hands as long as Dr. Robinson was around. In the military service he had regarded Bill as an affable, easy going individual who would simply turn things over to him if he came to Spokane. However, in the early post-war days it was not Bill's nature to be around things and not be involved. He had been too accustomed to making all the decisions himself in the pre-war years.

Schlicke was asked to see a patient at Sacred Heart for another of the "old gang" at the insistence of the family. The family was all present when the consultation took place and because Schlicke replied to a few of their questions he was called on the carpet by the Sister Superior and severely upbraided for this breach of ethics. A similar incident occurred at the Deaconess where he was obliged to assume the care of a young woman moribund from intestinal obstruction. After fluids and electrolytes had been restored and the obstruction relieved Schlicke received a call from the patient's former physician reminding him that he had come into the community under a cloud and that he wouldn't last long in Spokane if he persisted in activities of this type. Perhaps the most distressing incident of this sort occurred when Schlicke operated on a woman with a fecal fistula and removed a gauze sponge which had been left in the abdomen by her previous physician. When after her recovery there was talk of a law suit widespread obloquy was directed at Schlicke. What made this particularly painful was the fact that the original surgeon was one of the few doctors in Spokane who had gone out of his way to be friendly and who would be the last person in the world Schlicke would wish to damage. Calls were made on the President of the County Medical Society and other local dignitaries in the effort to explain that every effort had been made to protect the original doctor.

One of Schlicke's first cases at St. Luke's was that of an old man who walked into a crowded Montana saloon one night with a lighted stick of dynamite in each hand. "All of you sons of bitches better get out of here," he shouted, "I'm going to blow the place up!" Fortunately everyone did except the old man. Two days later someone poking through the rubble discovered him there and still breathing. He was now blind, deaf and had both hands blown off but amazingly, still alive. They bundled him into a plane and flew him to Spokane. There was little that could be done but tidy things up a bit, but incredibly it was several more days before the poor old fellow died.

In the early days all activities in the X-ray department on the lower floor of the Clinic were carried out by the chief and only technician. Occasionally the doctors would come down to observe fluoroscopic procedures and of course interpreted all of their own films. This obviously was a most unsatisfactory arrangement so Sharpe and Schlicke approached one of the larger X-ray firms to see if they could arrange for expert coverage. The meeting was held in the firm's office one Sunday morning and it ended up with the Clinic representatives being told that the firm could not risk its reputation by association with such a disreputable organization. These were bitter experiences for proud and well trained young men.

The physical arrangements at the Clinic were rather interesting. Patients walked in the front door. They were greeted by the receptionist who entered their names in a log book resting on a newel post at the foot of the main stairway. A counter was provided for this purpose at a later date. Drs. Sharpe and Robinson had their offices in the former dining room and study while Dr. Schlicke had taken over the Robinson bedroom. The pantry had been converted into a minor surgery room and the old kitchen was used for sigmoidoscopic examinations, the patients hanging their torsos over the end of a table and resting their heads on a foot stool. The laboratory was in a room adjacent to the kitchen and the X-ray equipment on the lowermost floor. The internists and others were up on the top floor.

The principle means of communication between the two floors was by shouting up and down the stairway.

8

EXPANSION AND ADDITIONS

BEFORE THE YEAR OF 1947 was over there had been three new additions to the staff and it was obvious that more space was needed. An eighteen foot easement on Dr. Robinson's property was obtained and a one story addition with twelve examining rooms was erected on the east side of the clinic building. It was originally planned to remove a huge lava outcropping which was in this area but as jack-hammers and power shovels after several days of expensive effort failed to dent the monolith and blasting was not allowed, the architect's plans were altered and the contractor, John Anderson, proceeded to build around it. The only disadvantage to the change was that the new addition to the laboratory was quite a bit narrower than had been anticipated.

The additions to the staff were Dr. Benjamin H. Inloes, Jr., an obstetrician and gynecologist from Maryland who arrived that summer and was soon admitted to the partnership. Dr. Samuel K. McIlvanie who came on as a salaried physician in August and left in June, 1948, for post-graduate training in hematology at the University of Louisville, and Dr. Harvey Gayle Copsey an internist from Broken Bow, Nebraska. Inloes hadn't been delivering babies for very long before he began talking of adding an associate to perform this chore so that he could devote more time to gynecologic surgery, a concept which did not sit too well with the other three surgeons, a good portion of whose operative load fell within this field. Dr. McIlvanie was a graduate of Washington State College who had earned a Master's degree at the University of Arizona and entered the U.S. Forest Service. He later earned an M.D. degree at the University of Louisville in 1946 and interned at the University of Pennsylvania Hospital. After completing his residency he returned to the Rockwood Clinic in 1950, only to leave again for a stint in the Army. He returned in November, 1952, this time to stay, becoming a partner in January, 1953. Dr. Copsey attended college and medical school at the University of Nebraska and interned at St. Joseph's Hospital in Kansas City, Missouri. He served a fellowship in internal medicine at the Mayo Clinic and then spent the next two years in the Army, most of this time on the neurological wards at Halloran General Hospital, Staten Island, New York. His two brothers were pilots in the Army Air Corps during World War Two and flew many combat missions, one in the European Theater of Operations and the other in the South Pacific. Before joining the Rockwood Clinic he had spent seven disillusioning months in practice with a general practitioner in Missoula, Montana. He became a partner in January, 1948.

In the meantime some rather complicated refinancing and business reorganization was taking place. Dr. Sharpe was anxious ultimately to achieve some sort of tripartite arrangement such as existed at the Mayo Clinic. Mayo's at that time was organized as the Mayo Clinic, the Mayo Foundation, and the Mayo Properties Association. The Foundation was created by a large personal donation of cash by the Drs. Mayo to the University of Minnesota. The income from this gift was to be for graduate medical and surgical instruction and research under the direction of the University. The Mayo Clinic was a voluntary association of physicians (not a corporation or partnership). Neither the associates nor their estates participated in any profits or liability of the enterprise which was managed by a Board of Governors. The Clinic was the operating arm of the institution which conducted the group practice of medicine. Any profits were fully taxable. The Mayo Properties Association was a charitable, benevolent, educational corporation with no stock outstanding which like the Foundation was started by funds and holdings of the Drs. Mayo. All buildings, equipment and records were owned by the Mayo Properties Association which rented these to the Clinic. Under a special act passed by the Legislature of Minnesota the Mayo Properties Association had the legal right to practice medicine and surgery under the name and style of Mayo Clinic, to study the causes of human ailments and to conduct research. No part of the net income or property, or of assets on dissolution should ever inure to the benefit of the members or any private individual. It was wholly exempt from paying federal or state income taxes. The Association and the Clinic were in a landlord-tenant relationship. The rental paid was the entire net income of the Clinic after settlement of obligations, expenses and the salaries of the staff. The Mayo Clinic was devoted to the care of the sick and any excess income above the fair and just compensation of the staff, should via the Mayo Properties Association, as a repository, be used solely in the fields of medical education and research.

This, with some notable exceptions was the general plan envisioned for the Rockwood Clinic. First when it became apparent that the Clinic had outgrown its facilities the Foundation sold the real estate to Drs. Robinson, Sharpe and Schlicke and their wives for the $58,828 therein invested, of which $23,787 had already been paid. The purchasers assumed a new mortgage for $32,000 and a note to Dr. Robinson for

$7738 and agreed to pay for this in monthly installments of $150 at 3% interest. A month later the purchasers signed a deed reconveying the property to the Robinson Foundation, following which it was sold back to the partners so as to include Dr. Delaney and his wife. A new mortgage for $50,000 was offered by the Aetna Life Insurance Company to discharge the old mortgage, finance the construction of the new wing and acquire the eighteen feet of the Robinson property. As the year drew to an end the purchasers assigned all of their rights over to the newly formed Rockwood Holding Corporation which was duly licensed by the Secretary of State and whose purpose was to take over the physical properties and contracts formerly owned by the partners along with all the furnishings and equipment. The Clinic Partnership then leased this whole complex from the Holding Corporation for $1500 a month. The Internal Revenue Service was watching all of these manipulations closely to see what happened to the funds held by the Foundation, and the State of Washington had its eye on the Holding Corporation since state laws at that time, in contrast to those of Minnesota, did not permit a corporation to engage in the practice of medicine. The lawyers and accountants were kept busy trying to avoid further tax problems.

Since there was no longer any interest in accumulating funds for rebuilding a hospital gradual dispersal of the Foundation's funds to various charitable causes was begun. C. Tod Oien and Lewis Klaue, the architect for the new wing were added to the Foundation Board of Trustees. The stockholders in the Holding Corporation at that time and the distribution of the 500 shares of capital stock subscribed by them were as follows: Robinson—40%, Sharpe—39%, Schlicke—16% and Delaney—5%.

The new wing was occupied in 1948 and proved quite satisfactory but it was soon found that the Holding Corporation could not operate efficiently at its present income so the rent was raised to $2100 a month retroactive to January 1, 1948. Later in the year shares of stock were sold to the partners at $100 a share. Robinson, Sharpe, Schlicke and Delaney each received twenty shares and Copsey ten. At Sharpe's suggestion, MacEachern was awarded a $550 bonus for the excellent job he was doing. The only addition to the staff this year was Dr. F. Robert Berghan a graduate of the University of Oregon Medical School. He had been in general practice in Toledo, Oregon, before coming to the Clinic. Applicants for staff positions usually came in reponse to requests directed by staff physicians to friends at institutions where they had trained or inquiries to medical procurement agencies. Less frequently they would simply show up at the front door. No one was quite sure how Berghan had found his way here but being a personable and capable young man he was hired. In 1949 he left for a residency in internal medicine at Henry Ford Hospital and a second tour of duty in the Navy which he was able to arrange so as to run concurrently. He returned in October of 1951 and became a partner in January, 1952, having as his subspecialty, endocrinology.

As the year drew to a close the first near medical disaster in the Clinic family occurred. Mary Lou Sharpe, who had borne her first child the first year she was in Spokane, was found in an unconscious state on the floor of her home. She was rushed to St. Luke's Hospital by ambulance arriving there in a state of profound shock with an imperceptible pulse. It was felt that she had a ruptured ectopic pregnancy so blood transfusions were started and she was taken to the operating room where Dr. Inloes, assisted by Schlicke and Dr. Richard McCartan, operated on her. A massive hemoperitoneum was evacuated and a right salpingo-oophorectomy carried out for a ruptured right tubal pregnancy and large follicular cyst of the ovary. Being a young and healthy woman she fortunately made an uneventful recovery and a year and a half later gave birth to her second son. It was, however, a terrifying experience for all concerned. Incidentally, earlier that year Hilda Schlicke had been operated on for a strangulated femoral hernia.

On the positive side the first professional recognition any of the post war doctors received occurred in 1948 when Schlicke was appointed chairman of the surgical committee at St. Luke's Hospital. This was indeed a welcome event in view of the generally hostile atmosphere throughout much of the community.

Dr. McCartan, who had assisted in the operation on Mrs. Sharpe, was then a surgical resident at St. Luke's where he had also been an intern. A native of Butte, Montana, he attended Carroll College in Helena and Medical School at Creighton University in Omaha. He was highly regarded by the Clinic men who had worked with him at St. Luke's and therefore invited to join them in 1949. He left for a two year stint in the Army in 1951, then returned and became a partner in January, 1954. Later in the year Dr. Arch H. Logan, Jr., whose father was an internist and his brother a pediatrician at the Mayo Clinic, came to work. He was a graduate of Washington and Jefferson College, earned his M.D. degree at Rush Medical School and interned at Geisinger Memorial Hospital in Danville, Pennsylvania. He completed a fellowship in internal medicine at the Mayo

Clinic with a three year interruption due to Army service. He became a partner in July of 1950.

When Dr. Logan and his wife, Virginia, moved to Spokane they drove out by car from Rochester. All of their more valuable possessions, such as silverware, cameras and so on, which they were reluctant to entrust to the commercial movers who were transporting their household furnishings, they brought with them personally in their car. The evening they arrived they spent with friends and when they prepared to leave their automobile had disappeared. It was later recovered but with all of their treasures stolen. This was indeed an inauspicious introduction to Spokane.

A great step forward toward higher quality work was taken in June when a contract was signed with Dr. Melvin Aspray to conduct the diagnostic radiology for the Clinic on a part time basis. He at least had no fear of contamination by such an association and the arrangement proved to be a happy one, continuing until the work load had increased to the extent that the Clinic took on a full time radiologist.

9

THE YEAR OF DECISION—1950

1950 TURNED OUT TO BE "The Year of Decision." Before it drew to a close the partners felt that if they were able to successfully weather the crises which it brought they could cope with any eventuality which the future might bring. It created a bond among the remaining partners which remains strong to this day. The year started out propitiously enough. In January the Trustees of the Foundation voted to donate $10,000 over a period of five years to St. Luke's Hospital which had treated them so well and which was now having serious financial problems. Dr. Delaney replaced Mr. Klaue on the Foundation Board and MacEachern replaced Tod Oien. A student loan was extended to Dr. McIlvanie. The west porch was enclosed and the space leased to Bert S. Densow, a local drug store owner to operate a pharmacy. This proved through the years to be a great convenience to patients, and to the Clinic as a source of pharmaceutical and other supplies. The first employee was John Platter, a most happy choice, although he had serious misgivings at the start, for the first winter was a monster. For at least two months very few patients could get to the Clinic and the pharmacy business was a disaster. Under these conditions the owner was glad his rental was 10% of his gross earnings and not a fixed sum. With the coming of spring business improved and has prospered ever since. John Anderson resigned from the Foundation Board. The Board decided to set up a $1000 research fund for the study of arteriosclerosis and collagen diseases when the money became available. Some new and expensive X-ray equipment was purchased.

Then came a law-suit. An obstetrical patient of Ben Inloes who suffered a post-partum hemorrhage, felt that her care had been improper and sued the Clinic and St. Luke's Hospital. Different insurance companies represented the two defendants and as a result each of them blamed the other for what had transpired. Finally a settlement was reached, a decision about which Inloes was allowed very little if anything to say. He felt that it was a reflection on his professional competence and would have preferred a vigorous defense. Adding to his unhappiness about this time was his wife's chronic disaffection with the Pacific Northwest and her nostalgia for the South. To everyone's distress he became the first partner to leave and left for Virginia and private practice. A separation agreement resulted in Inloes receiving $10,707 over a ten year period as his portion. It is regrettable to relate that he was unhappy with this as well, feeling that it should have been considerably more. There was also some difficulty getting him to release his shares in the Corporation, without which no changes in its structure or finances could take place.

But by far the most serious problem was that something was happening to Wendell Sharpe. As had been intended, Robinson had been gradually cutting back on his professional activities and spending more and more time away from the Clinic. As has been told, before the war it had been essentially a one man show. Minutes of the meetings of the stockholders in those days usually opened with, "Dr. Robinson addressed the members...." and that was pretty much it. In the new Clinic Sharpe was the director, manager, operator, and chief entrepreneur. For this he received $100 a month more than the $600 stipend of the other partners. Although there were frequent staff meetings they were essentially briefing sessions to inform the partners about decisions which he had made. Scrupulous minutes were kept of the Foundation and Holding Corporation meetings but none were kept of the Partnership meetings until October, 1950, when it had become obvious that an accurate record of the proceedings was essential. The everyday activities of the Clinic, the hiring and firing of professional and lay help, the distribution of profits and even advice in regard to the need for a larger home or a new car was handled by Sharpe. MacEachern was strictly his "leg man." Although his title varied from building superintendent to business manager, he was in reality a super errand-boy who had nothing to do with decisions or even the direction of the business office. Sharpe ran things in an authoritative manner, but at times Robinson from force of habit would order some building project, equipment or books or interfere in matters pertaining to personnel. Whenever this occurred Sharpe would be extremely upset.

Perhaps the first cause for concern was Sharpe's living standard. When he arrived he had no more financial resources than the other young partners, which were for the most part negligible. Yet shortly after he came to Spokane he acquired a magnificent home, a Cadillac Fleetwood sedan and maintained a life style which no one else could afford. One of the inducements held out to all potential partners was the concept of a wondrous cornucopia referred to as "accounts receivable." The actual value was always nebulous but it would always be there in seemingly unlimited amounts whenever needed. One of the deterrents against anyone leaving the partnership was that Sharpe insisted all interest in the accounts receivable would be forfeited. As it turned out, Robinson and

Sharpe were able to draw on these funds from time to time to meet personal expenses.

But even stranger things were happening. Sharpe began to be away from the Clinic with increasing frequency during the day. He explained these absences by the increasing demands on his time by outside consultations and operations at hospitals other than St. Luke's. Then he would spend untold hours late at night at the Clinic going over old records, writing voluminous notes and stapling pages together in the charts. He would also spend a lot of time riding around on unknown errands in his big Cadillac. One night the car turned up missing only to be found a block away undamaged. One memorable evening the Sharpes and the Schlickes were having dinner together at the Early Birds Club. This was an elegant establishment in the basement of the Davenport Hotel. Right after World War Two it was one of the few places where good beef was available and of course it was only at private clubs that one could buy liquor by the drink. The dining room was presided over by the genial maitre d', George Hespedis. The ever busy, then legal slot machines made it possible to secure food and first class music and entertainment at a price that fit the purses of impecunious young doctors. On this evening there was a comedian who had performed for the Mayo Unit in New Guinea. He had been happy to visit with an old acquaintance and in his next set he made a very flattering reference to the Rockwood Clinic in one of his gags which he thought would wow the audience. He never did understand why it fell so flat.

In the midst of dinner Sharpe suddenly disappeared only returning when the dancing was over and everyone was heading home. He explained that he had been called out to Fairchild Air Force Base where he was a consultant. Fairchild was an important Strategic Air Command Base on the outskirts of Spokane. It seemed that his expertise in handling prisoners of war had been needed because a planeload of Russian military personnel, some wounded, had been flown in. Everything was very hush-hush and mysterious. Poor old Schlicke was getting a terrible inferiority complex and even a little paranoia since there was so little demand for his services outside of the Clinic.

In point of fact even Sharpe's wife, Mary Lou, was getting worried and it was all too apparent to most of the partners that there was something decidedly abnormal about Sharpe's behavior. Schlicke who had known him for so long and made excuses for what had seemed like the slight idiosyncracies of genius through the years was the last to appreciate this fact. He finally became convinced when he called the operating suite where Sharpe supposedly had been working all afternoon on an extensive tendon repair and learned that no such operation had been performed that day and that Sharpe had not even been seen at the hospital. One or two other checks soon revealed that a number of other alleged events had simply never occurred. This was shattering news for now if one looked back, how was one to decide what had ever happened and what was pure fantasy? Moreover it was then discovered that Sharpe had been consuming huge quantities of amphetamines and barbiturates. In any event it was obvious that someone in this condition should not be seeing patients.

Schlicke and Delaney called on attorney Win Chandler who was a good friend and the current legal counselor for the Clinic. His advice was sought on how best to proceed and to determine what the Clinic's legal liability would be if an attempt was made to prevent Sharpe from working. Chandler was thunderstruck and could scarcely believe his ears. He had had a lot of business dealings with Sharpe in the reorganization of the Clinic's financial structure and had been greatly impressed by his brilliance. It was Chandler's opinion that if things truly were as they had been presented to him, the greatest liability to the Clinic lay in permitting Sharpe to continue practicing. The next day Sharpe's brother, a Federal Bureau of Investigation agent from Jackson, Michigan, appeared on the scene to see what was going on. Schlicke and he had previously met so the two of them went out to Eastern State Hospital where Dr. Robert Southcomb, a psychiatrist, was serving as Superintendent. He agreed that at the very least Sharpe needed psychiatric evaluation and probably treatment. He also had been a good friend and offered to do anything he could to help.

The first partnership minutes, dated October 18, 1950, tell of a traumatic meeting. Present were Robinson, Sharpe, Schlicke, Delaney, Copsey, Logan and MacEachern. Schlicke proposed that in view of Sharpe's physical condition he should be granted a four to six month's leave of absence during which period he should seek medical attention. Delaney urged Sharpe to seek this medical advice outside of the Clinic. Sharpe categorically rejected these suggestions and said he would prefer to sever all connections with the Clinic as of March 1, 1951. Robinson said that if this was his attitude his partnership connections should be severed immediately. Another meeting of the partners was held two days later. This time Sharpe did not attend. The partners' views regarding Sharpe were reiterated and it was unanimously agreed that until changed by a meeting of the partners, that as of that day, October 20, 1950, Sharpe was no longer to participate in any business concerning the Rockwood Clinic, either professionally or otherwise. A copy of the minutes of this meeting was taken to Sharpe at his home by MacEachern. Sharpe's response was that he was only interested in his original contract—the only one he had ever signed.

At the November meeting of the partners it was voted to continue Sharpe's drawing account during his leave of absence. In January, 1951, Sharpe announced by letter that he wished his severance dated April 1, 1951, but since he still refused to seek medical care the partners held out for December 31, 1950. Sharpe also claimed that $33,000 was due him from the accounts receivable. Arbitrators were appointed to work out a final settlement and after painstaking, delicate and understanding negotiations in which Mr. Chandler played a leading role an agreement was drawn up and signed by the parties involved, happily without the need for litigation. The final settlement contained the following stipulations:

1. Sharpe to release all rights and interest in the accounts receivable, if 10% of any part collected were given to MacEachern.
2. Sharpe to transfer his eighty-three shares of capital stock to the Rockwood Holding Corporation.
3. The Rockwood Clinic to pay Sharpe $11,500 and pay any outstanding bills in addition to the $2,700 he received subsequent to withdrawal from the Clinic.
4. The Clinic to relieve him of any personal responsibility in relation to the mortgage.
5. This was to be the final settlement with no further claims to be made by either party.

Mr. Chandler wrote, "This matter has involved attention and negotiation extending over a period of several months and was of extreme financial, professional and personal concern to the Clinic and its members. The settlement finally reached was, I think, a great deal better from the Clinic's standpoint than anyone would have expected."

After leaving Spokane Sharpe attempted practice in several settings with unhappy results, but finally became sufficiently readjusted to hold down a job at the Veterans' Hospital in Des Moines, Iowa, where with the sympathetic support of the Chief of Surgery, Dr. Louis Palumbo, he was able to work until his retirement in 1975. He then moved with his long suffering wife to Minneapolis where he resided until his death in 1978.

While all this was going on a replacement for Inloes was secured in the person of Dr. Llewelyn B. Harville. He had no sooner started work than in early November, 1950, while out duck hunting he sustained an anterior myocardial infarct, for which he was hospitalized. The myocardial damage was fortunately not great and his recovery rapid but it was problematical how much work he would be able to do. He resigned the following spring, moved to Richland and established a limited private practice. He had not been admitted to the partnership.

The only light touch in this otherwise dismal year was in the request of our chief receptionist, Mrs. Soderquist, to be replaced. She had always taken her work very seriously and one night while she and her husband were in bed he affectionately threw his arm over her. Coming half awake she mumbled, "Do you have an appointment?" This was enough as far as he was concerned and so to save their marriage the Clinic magnanimously granted her request.

The work load in the X-ray Department had increased greatly so Dr. Kenneth Gross, who had been working for Dr. Aspray and providing the Clinic with part time coverage, was approached about coming with the Clinic full time. He was interested but unfortunately prevented by the terms of his existing contract. The vulnerability of all the partners for further military service in view of the war in Korea led to the insertion of a new war clause in the partnership agreement and the increasing number of patients led to an intensified search for additional doctors. A prestigious firm of accountants, LeMaster and Daniels, was engaged to make an independent analysis of the Clinic's accounting system. Dr. Edward Turner, the dean of the University of Washington Medical School was contacted in regard to the possible placement of medical trainees at the Clinic for a year at a time. Repeated changes in laboratory personnel had taken place and Miss Mary Ann Ripple agreed to head up its operation after the first of the new year.

As the year drew to a close, an athletic young physician named Richard H. Hempstead, who was a urologic fellow at the Mayo Clinic and whose father was a nose and throat specialist on the staff there came to look over the Rockwood Clinic. He was a graduate of Dartmouth and the University of Michigan and interned at Alameda County Hospital in Oakland, California. At a reception one evening, Mrs. Delaney, who took a great interest in such matters began to interrogate him regarding his private life and family. She found out that he was a bachelor, had a sister-divorced, and a brother-unmarried, whereon she inquired, "Goodness, isn't anyone in your family married?" Hempstead innocently replied, "Yes.

my father and mother are." Fortunately by the time he came to work at the Clinic a year later he had extricated himself from this anomalous position by acquiring a bride, an artistic young lady named Alice Hagen. Except for an eleven month recall into the Navy in 1953, he has been the Clinic urologist ever since.

10

MORE OF THE FATEFUL FIFTIES

THE REMAINING CLINIC PARTNERS formed a very close knit group. They were not only professional colleagues but close personal friends. They did much of their socializing together, often gathering on Saturday nights at one of their homes for music, dancing and refreshments. For a while there was a Santa Claus who visited the children at Christmas time and for fourteen years the clan gathered at the Schlickes' for New Year's Eve. Sunday morning there was a car pool to get the children to Sunday school and often on Sunday afternoons home visits were exchanged. Everyone, except Robinson, regardless of specialty took his turn as the doctor on call. Requests for house calls were frequent and almost always responded to, often leading to humorous, bizarre or sometimes even sad experiences in a very different environment from the impersonal surroundings of a hospital emergency room. If the patient required hospitalization this was arranged and the appropriate specialist who would be on second call, notified. If the problem could be handled on an out-patient basis an appointment was arranged with the doctor in whose field the problem lay. It was essentially triage, first aid and basic primary care.

Some of the house calls were simply a nuisance such as when spoiled, well heeled patients who had had too much to drink suffered little cuts or bruises and demanded immediate attention on the spot. But there were other kinds. Schlicke remembers going to the home of a lady upon whom he had performed an exploration of the common bile duct. Her T-tube had stopped draining so he attempted to irrigate it. The simple procedure was made difficult by the attentions of the lady's dog which kept snapping at his heels. There was the man whose wound broke down after an operation for sarcoma of the parotid who was lying cheerfully in bed at home while his wound was swarming with maggots; the lady sitting stone dead on her toilet where she had suffered a heart attack; the lady with an enormous ovarian cyst which had become twisted and was causing great pain, who waited until late at night to call so that she would not attract the attention of her nosy neighbors, and then the ambulance which had been summoned to take her to the hospital roaring up with lights flashing and siren wailing.

Joe Delaney used to tell about treating a young lady in what turned out to be a brothel operated by a Chinese madam who pulled a fruit jar stuffed with five and ten dollar bills out from under the bed to pay him. Then there was the night Bill Anderson, the Clinic's newest doctor, was called down to a house in Peaceful Valley. Bill wondered why he had been called since Joe was the doctor on duty. More than this he wondered whether it would be safe to go in since it was very dark, very quiet and a spooky looking place. As he walked up with considerable trepidation to knock on the door, the door was flung open and out marched Joe who had gotten the call after all.

There was the telephone call from a lady whose husband had had a gastric resection who requested a house call because he was having some wound drainage. She was advised to take him to the Clinic since this was during the middle of the day. She persisted, however, so the reluctant surgeon agreed to drop by. When he arrived the patient was standing on his front steps holding a saturated bath towel which contained an incredible number of loops of small bowel. "For God's sake get back in the house" cried the astonished surgeon, "You'll ruin my reputation!" When he reentered his home the man continued to stand. He was admonished to lie down on the sofa until an ambulance could be called. He averred that he felt better standing up. "That's fine" said the surgeon, "but I'd feel much better with you lying down." Happily he made an uneventful recovery after the repair of his wound disruption.

Perhaps one of the most memorable incidents followed a call from an intern at a hospital where the group seldom worked to see his wife who was ill. Schlicke pulled up before a new ranch style home and was admitted by a well dressed pleasant young couple who said they were looking after things and caring for the two children until the doctor returned. Everyone sat in the living room and chatted politely until that time. The young doctor upon his arrival conducted the surgeon to the master bedroom. It was a shambles. The walls were smudged and blood stained. Shattered pictures littered the floor. A broken lamp and tube of contraceptive jelly were on a battered bedside table. On the bed lay a totally unconscious young woman. It was hard to tell what she might have looked like because her face was so battered and swollen. Her eyelids were swelled shut and blackened, her lips puffy and cut. Her head had been completely shaved. There was blood about her nose and lips and on the bedding. Aside from this there seemed to be no other injuries except multiple bruises. The obvious question was, "What on earth happened to her?" the answer, "We had an argument." "When?" "Two days ago." "Has she had any care?" "No, but she's better now." "She must be taken to the hospital." "That would mean my ruin." "Her death will ruin you far more." A compromise was reached whereby whatever could be done at home would be for the next few hours but if there was not decided improvement she either went to the hospital or the police would be notified. A few hours elapsed, there was no change in her condition so she was moved to a hospital where appropriate studies and treatment could be carried out. As long as everything turned out satisfactorily the cause of her problems would be listed as an automobile accident. As it turned out, aside from a severe cerebral contusion from which she made a complete recovery and the assorted cuts, abrasions and bruises and a broken nose there were no serious injuries uncovered. After a few days she was sent home, quite satisfied with the way things had been managed. Her mother had arrived from out of town to help care for the patient and her children and was most appreciative. No one seemed upset with the husband. An interesting sequel occurred a few months later at the time of the State Medical Association meeting in Seattle. Schlicke and his wife were walking out of the front door of the Olympic Hotel when they were greeted effusively by a happy family group who happened to be standing there. There were no reminiscences, just a brief period of cheery chit-chat. The past seemed to have been forgotten. Maybe it was an automobile accident?

There was the retired gunsmith whose wife developed a malignant tumor of her lower bowel. The husband blandly informed the consulting surgeon that he would shoot him if he performed a colostomy on his wife. Fortunately this proved not to be necessary and she made a good recovery from the removal of her tumor. A few days after she returned home from the hospital the poor woman was shot to death by her deranged husband. A few minutes later he was involved in a minor traffic accident. At that time the police concerned themselves with such matters even though there was no bodily injury involved. By so doing they found him to be carrying a loaded pistol and learned of the murder. When they asked him where he thought he was going, he replied, "The Rockwood Clinic." It is not pleasant to contemplate what might have happened had he not been involved in a little fender bending.

After these lugubrious tales it probably would be prudent to conclude these house call reminiscences with something in a lighter vein. There was one family in Spokane which had made Schlicke's life miserable with frequent demands for nocturnal visits. Each time one of them called their frantic appeals made it sound as though someone in the family, usually mother, was in dire straits, although from previous experience, it was almost certain to prove a false alarm after the doctor arrived. He had pretty much reached the limit of his patience and vowed never to set foot in their home again when he was awakened from his slumbers one night to be told that the daughter was critically ill with abdominal pain. Schlicke was sure it would be just another useless outing, but since the daughter seemed to be the one sensible member of the family he agreed to come over. When he arrived at the house he was immediately escorted to her bedroom where she was found to be writhing about with an acute irritable bowel syndrome precipitated by a family squabble. After he had assured himself that there was nothing seriously wrong with the girl he gave vent to his indignation in no uncertain terms. The whole family was told what he thought of them and their constant and unreasonable demands on his time. How, he inquired, was he supposed to render adequate care to the remainder of his patients if he was up all night on wild goose chases which robbed him of his well earned rest? When he finished his tirade he picked up his bag, clapped his hat on his head and stormed to the nearest door in high dudgeon, flung it open and marched out of the room into the clothes closet. Since this devastating blow to his dignity he has never worn a hat.

Of course humiliating experiences are not restricted to house calls but may occur in the operating room as well. Schlicke was operating on a lady with peritonitis under spinal anesthesia. Her problem proved to be due to a toothpick which she had swallowed and which had perforated her small intestine. Schlicke was expounding eruditely to his assistant about this unusual condition when from beyond the anesthesia screen came the patient's voice protesting that he must be mistaken since she was edentulous, wore full dentures and had no need for toothpicks. An unseemly argument was only prevented by the surgeon reaching across the screen and pushing the toothpick in front of her face. She then admitted to having eaten a piece of birthday cake, the layers of which had been held together by toothpicks. On another occasion he was carrying out an operation for varicose veins on a meat cutter, again under spinal anesthesia which for obvious reasons he seldom uses any more. As one of the veins was extracted the end of the vein stripper described an arc through the air and splattered blood beyond the anesthesia screen. The surgeon peered over the screen and watched the anesthetist wiping the blood off the patient's face. Deeply embarassed he apologized profusely to the patient, who replied, "Oh, that's all right Doc, I'm a butcher myself."

* * * * * * *

Far from feeling defeated as they moved into the new year, the partners at their initial meeting in 1951 began discussing the need for another story on the new wing. Preliminary architectural plans were prepared, at which point Delaney protested that he had not given his consent. The Holding Corporation was never the less able to borrow $65,000 over fifteen years at 4½% from the Aetna Life Insurance Company to finance the addition and take over the old mortgage. In order to do this the Corporation had to acquire the title to the real estate, but after consummation of the new mortgage the Corporation was to reconvey the premises to the Foundation and execute with it a new contract of purchase on the same terms as the unpaid balance of the present contract. By the end of August the new addition was completed by Al Arsenault and his A.A.A. Construction Company making thirteen more examining rooms available. Anton Woodruff was the architect. The rent was raised from $2,000 to $2,500 a month and $15,000 more was borrowed at 6% interest from the First National Bank of Spokane to complete the improvements and obtain additional equipment, placing a chattel mortgage on the Clinic's X-ray equipment in order to accomplish this. Interestingly enough, with all these manipulations the original sales agreement of October 16, 1947, remained in full force.

Because of the added burden placed on Schlicke by the departure of Sharpe he was relieved of the responsibility of working up new patients, which had previously been done by all of the partners on a rotation or request basis. Schlicke was delighted when one day in the Sacred Heart operating suite he was approached by Dr. Thomas C. Wilder offering to make himself available as a replacement for Sharpe. Tom was a general surgeon who had completed a surgical fellowship at the Mayo Clinic and served as first assistant to Dr. Claude Dixon. His father, a world renowned expert on diabetes and nutrition was an internist on the staff of the Mayo Clinic, the author of a book on diabetes and the first to describe the disease state of hyperinsulinism. Tom had had an exciting career with the Navy in the South Pacific, after a brief tour of duty at Farragut Naval Base in Idaho. Since then he had been in solo practice in Spokane. That a man with this background and of this caliber should seek the Clinic out was a great morale boost to the group. Tom Wilder joined the group in April. His wife, Jean, was the daughter of Dr. Lillie, the head of the Ear, Nose and Throat Department at the Mayo Clinic. They had four sons, three of whom became physicians.

One evening the Wilders had planned a cocktail party in honor of a visiting friend. When the Schlickes arrived, early as usual, Jean asked Schlicke to serve as bartender. When he inquired where Tom was, Jean said he was down at the police station bailing out two of his boys who had been apprehended while tossing rocks through the window panes of their grammar school which was closed for the summer. Amazingly Jean was quite unruffled and able to function as a gracious and unperturbed hostess.

In the summer of 1951, Ralph Dean Luther joined the staff. A graduate of Jefferson Medical College, and a superbly trained orthopedist, he had worked with Dr. J.R. Moore at the Shriners' Hospital in Philadelphia and then spent several years in the Army, most of the time in Panama. Dean was a great asset to the Clinic, always in the foreground of his specialty in Spokane. He brought with him his wife, Mary, who was also a physician, and their daughter, Joan.

The following month, William E. Anderson, who had served an internship and one year surgical residency at Sacred Heart Hospital was hired to help out and to gain additional experience at the Rockwood Clinic. Bill had attended Jefferson Medical College. On his way to Spokane, he drove his car and brought with him his new bride, Doris, a nurse from Hershey, Pennsylvania. Bill was born and raised in Missoula, Montana and was an avid and skilled hunter and fisherman. He helped earn his way through Montana State College by working summers for the Forest Service as a smoke jumper. He had also done a tour of duty as a gob on the Battleship *Missouri*. On the way West he regaled Doris with stories to illustrate how wild and woolly it really was. One Sunday morning while driving across Montana they pulled up at an oasis called the Leaky Roof Saloon. Bill ordered a shot of whiskey and Doris thought she would like a "Coca Cola, please." The incredulous bartender stared at her and in his gravelly voice exclaimed, "Jesus Christ, lady, this is a saloon, not a God damn drug store."

A fourth addition to the staff this summer was Dr. John R. Tobin. He had attended Notre Dame and then received his M.D. degree from the University of Chicago Medical School, interning at Chicago's Presbyterian Hospital. During World War Two he served with the Fifth Infantry Division in the Italian campaign. He was an old friend of Arch Logan's and had also taken a fellowship in internal medicine at the Mayo Clinic. He and his wife, Peggy, were both expert golfers. John was never completely happy in private practice even though arrangements were made for him to carry out experimental research at Gonzaga University after he had become a partner. He resigned from the partnership in 1954, remaining as an employee until June, 1955, when he returned to the University of Chicago Medical School working at the Hektoen Institute for Medical Research. He also spent some further time at the Mayo Clinic doing post-graduate work in cardiology. Ultimately he devoted himself entirely to academic medicine and became Professor of Medicine at Loyola University Medical School. His withdrawal from the Clinic was relatively painless as everyone was so fond of John and Peggy that above all they wished to see them happy. A warm friendship was never affected by the change of course.

The time had come, it was decided, when full time X-ray coverage was needed, initially to be supplied by Aspray and Gross. A gastroscope which Sharpe had ordered but never used was turned over to the Foundation and then donated to the University of Washington Medical School. The agreement with MacEachern that he was to receive a portion of the accounts receivable was found to be too cumbersome so this was changed so as to give him a fixed percent of the net income as long as he was an employee of the Clinic. To ease the pain of buying into the corporation for $5,000 it was decided to withhold 50% of each partner's dividend from the Medical Service Bureau, Old Age Assistance and Welfare programs as a contribution to the Holding Corporation to be used for the purchase of equipment, property and building. By this time the partners' drawing accounts had risen to $900 a month with the exception of Robinson who received $1000. New trainees were getting $500 a month instead of the previous $350 to $400. It was also voted to start accumulating funds the following year to be used to pay off retiring partners. A new partnership agreement was drawn up and signed which contained a modified war clause and a restrictive clause where by any withdrawing partner was prohibited from practicing in Spokane County for two years.

A most important decision was the vote to continue the association of the Rockwood Clinic with the Medical Service Bureau although it persisted in denying any reimbursement for laboratory or X-ray work done at the Clinic. There had been several very unpleasant conferences between representatives of the Clinic and the Bureau Trustees. Dissatisfaction with the Bureau was becoming more widespread in the community, particularly among the internists, so in the hope that reforms would be forthcoming and to avoid the loss of the 20-25% of the Clinic patients who were Bureau subscribers the decision was made to maintain the association for a little longer trial.

The report of the study of the operation and methods of the business office by LeMaster and Daniels had not been flattering. Robinson suggested that a certified public accountant be sought to take over the duties of business manager, a job which with the growth of the Clinic had gone far beyond the capacities of MacEachern. A search was instituted and the Clinic was indeed fortunate in securing the services of Arch L. Jenkins, Jr. although he was not a C.P.A. In October of 1951 he assumed the role of business manager. This, at least was his title and he was an expert at this job, but he soon became so much more than that—friend, advisor, mediator, father confessor, trouble shooter and wet nurse to the often temperamental doctors. Above all, the "Coach," as he was affectionally called, was a team player and a loyal and proud member of the organization of which he was such an integral part. Born in North Carolina, he came to Spokane in 1925. After graduating from Lewis and Clark High School he went to Stanford where he received a degree in economics and journalism. He had edited the Lewis and Clark student paper and was the editor of the Stanford Daily. He entered the Army as an enlisted man in 1942 and emerged as a captain at the end of the war, having had twenty-two months of combat duty in Italy. After the war he went into the food manufacturing business with his father-in-law and later was the office manager for an insurance firm. Like other members of the team he had some misgivings at first. When he told a physician friend where he had accepted a job, the comment was, "Not that place!" One evening he attended a meeting of the Spokane Corral of the Westerners with Schlicke. A former high school vice principal of his inquired of Schlicke what Arch was doing now. When told, he said, "Too bad, I always thought he would amount to something." Arch served with finesse, faithfulness and great ability, ultimately bringing the Clinic into the computer age. He retired on September 30, 1977, after twenty-six years of service.

Once again there were concerns about the tax status of the Rockwood Holding Corporation. The Internal Revenue Service was closely scrutinizing small or personal holding corporations. Serious consideration was given to the possibility of either turning the Corporation over to the partnership or of transferring the title to its assets to the University of Washington. Several discussions actually were held with representatives of the University. It was finally decided that there would be little financial or tax advantage or relief of liability and distinct disadvantages as far as future expansion was concerned so these avenues of exploration were dropped. Finally, as of December 31, 1951, the Holding Corporation was dissolved and the Rockwood Holding Company, a co-partnership formed.

Robinson, who at this time was having far more trouble with his heart disease than most of the partners realized, was authorized to withdraw as much as he wished from active practice and ultimately to retire, while retaining his full salary and interest in the partnership earnings for as long as he lived. In addition to his heart problem he was suffering from frequent attacks of gout. Yet a third problem which was becoming a matter of increasing concern to his wife was the amount of medication he was consuming. His chief contribution to the Clinic at this time was his still not inconsiderable drawing power. Some of his more solvent patients at times created an annoying problem. They had been highly pampered in bygone days when, as Bill used to put it, they were "paying the freight" in the form of significantly increased charges. Now they were covered by prepaid insurance or the Medical Service Bureau and still expected the same type of privileged attention. At one point Delaney suggested that "undesirable patients be referred to someone else in the Clinic or outside of the Clinic altogether." No vote has been recorded in regard to this idea. Robinson still participated in the professional meetings when he was in town and not otherwise occupied. On one memorable evening he astonished the partners by giving an erudite and highly sophisticated presentation on steroid hormones and drugs, facilely diagraming their molecular structure on a black board as he went along.

The past year had been one of rapid transition. One of the changes which took place was a shift of hospital orientation from St. Luke's to Sacred Heart Hospital. St. Luke's had treated the staff of the Rockwood Clinic very well but the proximity of Sacred Heart just across the street was a convenience too great to be ingnored. Everyone on the staff was very busy and there was no question but that it was far more efficient and resulted in closer physician supervision of patients to have them nearby. Moreover Sacred Heart had softened its attitude toward the young men at the Rockwood Clinic and was in a stage of professional growth with the addition of top flight people to the supporting services such as pathology and radiology. Its surgical department had been significantly strengthened and its work was being subjected to careful and impartial monitoring. The orientation of the Rockwood Clinic toward Sacred Heart Hospital was the beginning of a very happy relationship which has continued up to the present.

At the same time it seemed as though there was always someone interested in having clinic doctors work outside of the Clinic. Delaney was invited to become a consulting cardiologist to the Veterans' Administration Hospital in Walla Walla. And then there were opportunities to take over other health facilities as satellite clinics in Colfax and Deer Park. At a later date our radiologists did briefly try to cover the hospital at Coulee Dam. All this was flattering but totally impractical.

In 1952 attorney William Bantz was engaged on a retainer fee as the Clinic's lawyer. He later became United States District Attorney and also a candidate for the United States Senate. His replacement was a highly regarded tax attorney, Paul Castoldi. The lease on the pharmacy was transferred to John Platter following the death of Bert Densow.

It was soon realized that if there was to be any further expansion that additional land would be needed. The Holding Company proceeded to purchase for $18,000 from Dr. Robinson the apartment building just north of the Clinic at West 49 Seventh Avenue where Inloes and MacEachern had been living and a year later purchased Dr. Robinson's residence just east of the Clinic for $20,000. Unsuccessful attempts were made to acquire the rooming house west of the Clinic operated by Mary Gianetsas. When the entirely new Sacred Heart Medical Center was erected about sixteen years later the main patient tower had to be built northward down the hill instead of east and west along the bluff to the south because Mrs. Gianetsas still refused to give up her property for an offer ten times as large as the one the Clinic had made.

A new partnership agreement was signed with a percentage of profit distribution as follows: Robinson, Schlicke, Delaney—18.5%, Copsey—17.5%, Logan—11.0%, Wilder—7.0%, Tobin, Berghan, Luther—4.0%. The partners voted to close the Clinic on Wednesday and Saturday afternoons keeping a skeleton staff on duty to cover emergencies. Rental paid by the Clinic to the Holding Company was set at $1,500 a month. Election to partnership included automatic admission to the Holding Company. The 50% contributed through retainage as working capital was to be of no value to them and not to be repaid on death or retirement. Partners who had already contributed were exempt from further contribution. The willingness to adopt such an arrangement by a group of doctors often personally strapped financially indicated the intensity of their commitment to the Clinic and their desire to have it grow and prosper.

In the amenities department it was voted to discontinue the previous practice of the Clinic sending Christmas cards to patients and to offer no professional discount for medical services rendered to chiropractors. The wearing of white gowns by physicians was left to the individual doctor's taste. A motion to set the retirement age of partners at 65 was passed with the option to continue on a salary basis without voting power or partnership responsibilities. Initially this option was entirely up to the retiring partner. In 1956 this was altered so as also to require the approval of a majority of the remaining partners and so arranged that it could be terminated at any time at the will of 75% of the partners. New doctors were to serve two years before being admitted to partnership. After the first year they were to receive the same basic salary as partners. After the second year they were to receive a negotiable percent of the profits. Full equality in total income with senior partners was to be achieved after seven years. The Clinic meanwhile was paying for car expenses, medical society dues, journal subscriptions, clinical trips and malpractice insurance. The equal distribution system has been a source of amazement to outsiders, yet it has made it possible to attract first class doctors and keep them happy. The feeling was that if after an initial probation period a new doctor was deemed worthy of partnership, as long as to the best of his ability he carried his share of the work load he should ultimately share equally in the profits as well as in the responsibilities and risks. Complex point formulas in some merit or incentive systems have proved to be the rocks on which more than one clinic has foundered. At about this same time the decision was reached to form an executive committee to assist and advise the business manager. It was to be composed of one surgeon, one internist and a third member selected from among the younger partners by the first two. The business manager was to serve as the permanent secretary of the committee.

The member having served the longest became chairman and also presided at the monthly partnership meetings. Members were to serve staggered six month terms for a maximum of three. It was felt wise to have a system of fairly rapid rotation in order to give all of the partners a feeling of participation and to familiarize them with the business workings of the Clinic rather than establishing an all powerful, semi-permanent Board of Governors. The original partners had become highly sensitized to autocracy and treasured the opportunity for expression and involvement afforded by the "town hall" type meetings of the entire partnership. If the Clinic continues to grow it is quite possible that the equal distribution system may have to be altered and the present type of meeting and decision making discarded as impractical and unwieldy and operation of the Clinic turned over to an enlarged and strengthened Board of Governors. But in these early and post-traumatic days universal involvement was essential and has continued to work surprisingly well, if not with maximum efficiency, up to the present. Through the years the minutes often record the same motions being made and the same endless arguments being conducted over and over again, but this is democracy and it has kept people happy.

A student loan was extended to Berghan as it had been to McIlvanie. A new partnership agreement was approved with sharing as follows: Robinson, Schlicke, Delaney and Copsey—15.1%, Logan—12.2%, Wilder, Tobin, Luther and Berghan—5.3%, McIlvanie and Hempstead—3.1%. Copsey and Logan were elected to the Board of Trustees of the Foundation and Jenkins replaced Onstine as a member and as its Secretary-Treasurer. Carl Nicholson, C.P.A. was engaged as the accountant for the Clinic. One of the first reforms accomplished under his guidance was the abolition of the pernicious practice of attempting to apportion specific amounts of the accounts receivable to individual doctors. As Jenkins has pointed out, "In a multi-specialty clinic with many ancillary services also producing revenues, it is really not possible to say which unpaid bill is the property of what doctor." It is startling to note that there is still $21,000 of such distributions carried on the Clinic books as "Goodwill" as a means of accounting for previous abuses of the system. Also there was to be accurate documentation of any expenses for which the doctors sought remuneration. Jenkins' insistence on strict enforcement of this regulation for everyone led to somewhat strained relations between him and the Robinsons. The agreement with MacEachern was changed so as to pay him a salary commensurate with his duties. The trouble was that it was becoming increasingly difficult to determine exactly what those duties were. He was not of much help to Jenkins in the business office. He had had considerable experience as a surgical technician when he was in the Army Medical Corps and since the Clinic's surgeons often needed extra help in the operating room it was suggested that this would be a valuable activity in which he could become involved. He refused even to discuss this, seeming to feel this was beneath the dignity of an executive. As a result it became necessary for the Clinic to engage the services of the first of a series of "scrub nurses."

In 1953 increased efforts were made to reduce the Foundation holdings by donations to such organizations as the Retail Trade Bureau, the Chamber of Commerce, the Municipal League, the Lilac Festival,

American Red Cross and the March of Dimes. A research committee was appointed to approve experimental and investigative projects and to maintain a diagnostic cross index file. The surgical department had started keeping a log of operative procedures several years earlier which had been a great help in the preparation of talks and papers and the review of work, but not until the introduction of computer facilities in the business office many years later was such an activity universally established throughout the Clinic.

Later this year when McCartan returned from his Army duty there was talk of setting up a Department of General Practice with him as chief and Dr. Anderson on his return from his second tour of duty in the Navy to be the first addition to the department. The idea, however, never caught on, the feeling being that primary care was already being satisfactorily provided by the internists. McCartan was invited to stay, but not as a partner. This decision was subsequently changed and he was admitted to the partnership in 1954. In 1955 he was sent to Chevalier Jackson's endoscopy clinic in Philadelphia for post graduate work in this field in which he developed great competence. Once the decision was definitely reached not to have a department of general practice it was hard to see where Bill Anderson would fit in and Schlicke had the difficult task of passing on this news to him. He left the following year and set up a highly successful solo general practice in the Spokane Valley and happily has remained a good friend.

The partners voted to have the Clinic associate itself with the American Association of Medical Clinics, now called the American Group Practice Association. Checks which the internists received for interpreting E.C.G.s were contributed to the Clinic Library fund.

Applications for the position of radiologist to the Clinic finally began to come in and in September a mutual temporary association agreement was signed with Dr. John Bartness to assume this position. He was to receive $900 a month and became a partner in 1955, if this proved mutually agreeable, which unfortunately it didn't. Drs. Aspray and Gross kindly agreed to supervise Bartness until he could take his State Licensing Board basic science examination and legally practice independently. To everyone's distress when that time arrived he flunked the examination, the only time this has ever happened to any addition to the staff. This created unanticipated difficulties and he was only able to continue working due to the willingness of Aspray and Gross to continue what had been planned as short term coverage and the agreement by Dr. Robert Rotchford the chairman of the State Board of Medical Examiners to approve the arrangement until the next examination was given. His eligibility for partnership was made contingent on his passing the examination. Other problems arose. He refused to submit to the physical examination which traditionally was carried out on all new employees and annually thereafter on partners. He wished to carry on part time work outside of the Clinic and in general resisted all regulations which the group had found it necessary to require for its survival. He had only minimal rapport with the staff and obviously should never have attempted to participate in group practice. He left the following summer and when last heard from was giving judo and karate lessons to a church group in a small town in southern Minnesota. After his departure Drs. Augustus Galloway and Drummond Sweeny came to the rescue by doing the radiologic work until a replacement for Bartness could be found.

11

SO YOU WANT A NEW BUILDING?

IT WAS IN FEBRUARY 1953 that the first formal discussion took place regarding the possible construction of a new building designed from the start as a medical clinic. It was agreed to finance the travel of Mr. John Dawson, a representative of Ellerbe and Company in St. Paul, the architects for the Mayo Clinic, for preliminary discussions and advice. The greatest concern was how an undertaking of such magnitude could be financed. It was heartening to hear Mr. Dawson's assurance, "If you really need a new building and want it badly enough, you will get it." George Nichols, a local real estate operator was invited to the next partnership meeting to talk over possible sites. Many were considered, some were too expensive, some had no room for parking, others had unlimited room for parking but were inconveniently located. It was ultimately agreed to concentrate on the general area in which the Clinic currently was located because of the character of the neighborhood, its proximity to two major hospitals and the availability of nearby public transportation. Within a year the property at West 312 Eighth Avenue, on the northwest corner of the junction with Bernard Street was purchased by the Rockwood Holding Company and Ellerbe and Company retained to conduct preliminary studies. Two members of the executive committee, Schlicke and Delaney, along with Mr. Jenkins, were sent to Great Falls, Montana to look over the new Great Falls Clinic building which Ellerbe had designed. They were highly pleased by what they saw and brought back many ideas which were helpful in the planning of the new Rockwood Clinic building. At the same meeting that the trip to Great Falls was authorized the Clinic rent was raised from $1,500 to $2,000 a month although there was no direct connection between this and the expenses incurred in the trip. After the sale of their home Dr. and Mrs. Robinson remained in residence paying $75 a month rent. Drs. Berghan, Schlicke and Delaney were chosen to serve as a building committee.

The greatest obstacle in the way of realization of the dream of a new building was where the money was to come from. Initial flights of fancy nurtured hopes of finding an "angel" who would leap at the opportunity to underwrite such a worthy community asset. As it turned out, among those consulted only one was seriously interested, but even he would only consider a multipurpose structure, built to his specifications. From the

Clinic's standpoint this would represent a scant improvement, except in size, over the improvised quarters previously occupied and any future alterations or expansion would be subject to the "angel's" whims. From his standpoint, or course, it would seem like sensible insurance since such a building would be designed so that it could be converted into an apartment or office building if the medical partnership fell on its face.

Members of the building committee met with numerous bankers and financiers. Jenkins and Schlicke well remember a luncheon at the Spokane Club with one of these august representatives from the lofty world of high finance. After a presentation of the Clinic's needs and desires and the banker's ascertaining that the Clinic had virtually no resources except its heavily mortgaged properties and the professional competence and integrity of the partnership, he commented, sententiously, "Many people would like to have a nice new building," and that was the end of that. The Clinic was even stuck with the bill for feeding the big stuffed shirt. In time, however, rumors began to circulate that the Spokane and Eastern Branch of the Seattle First National Bank was truly interested in helping promising ventures to develop. The Bank appeared to believe that such efforts were beneficial for the involved communities and that human resources, as exemplified by people of enterprise and ability, might have some value and be worth taking a chance on. As things began to look more hopeful in this direction and some preliminary assurances were received, the partners in their final act of 1953 voted to make the "S and E" Bank the depository for all Clinic funds. When the vice-president of the bank which previously had handled all of the Clinic's banking needs was apprized of the switch he called up to inquire why this had occurred. When the reason was explained, he asked if his bank had been given the opportunity to look into the matter and was assured that his bank had been the first one approached. This ended the conversation.

When he completed his internship at Sacred Heart Hospital in the summer of 1954 Dr. Jay Johnson was engaged at $400 a month, as a temporary addition to the staff. This was the last of a series of young doctors taken on before formal post graduate training. Although the idea was that they were to help out wherever needed they always ended up delivering primary care at the Clinic and were of little help to the other departments. It worked out well enough in the case of Drs. McIlvanie and Berghan but in other instances it failed to accomplish what had been intended. Perhaps if the Clinic had gone the route of setting up a department of general practice the arrangement would have been more satisfactory. Jay did a good job while he was with the Clinic and at the end of a year went to Duke University to take a residency in plastic surgery, but soon switched to urology. After completing his training in this field he returned to Spokane and has had a successful career as a solo practitioner in urology. Since that time the Clinic has only added men to the staff who have completed specialty training. Along the way in the past there had been other doctors who had worked at the Clinic for short periods of time while they made up their minds where and how they wished to practice. Dr. Hugh Brown, another internist named Peck and Charles Smick, a general practitioner, fell into this category.

At the beginning of this year a new partnership agreement had been signed so as to admit Dr. McCartan. It was agreed that Dr. Robinson would be exempted from the mandatory retirement rule and that there would be no terminal reimbursement for any partner who withdrew on his own initiative. A wise decision was made that all major proposals or projects were first to be reviewed by the executive committee before presentation to the partnership and then held over until the following partnership meeting before a final decision was made. The starting salary for new potential partners was increased to $700 a month, to be raised to $900 at six months with participation in profit sharing to start after one year and equality to be reached after a total of seven years. On the eve of his departure Dr. Tobin suggested that yearly adjustments of the partners' percentages should be decided by secret poll, the results to be determined by an outside accountant. With this type of thinking it was felt that he had made a wise decision in returning to academic medicine. At the last meeting of the year it was reported that the three senior partners had met with Dr. Robinson to discuss his withdrawal from practice and formal retirement. His participation in the profits was to be reduced by 50% as of the first of the next year. His health was deteriorating, he was spending very little time at the Clinic which, of course, was in accord with former agreements, but the greatest cause for concern was that the quality of his work was falling off appreciably. In the Scrooge department it was voted to have a full crew on duty all day on Christmas eve and on New Year's Eve.

Throughout this year the building committee had been most active. City codes and restrictions were studied to determine whether rezoning would be necessary in connection with the new building. Sacred Heart Hospital was approached to determine whether it was interested in purchasing the present Clinic property. It was not. In March the purchase of the lot at Eighth and Bernard had been formally authorized. The building committee was told to offer the owners between $50,000 and $60,000 and to find out if the Culmstock Lodge just north of the Culmstock Arms on Washington Street could be obtained. The apartment building at West 49 Seventh Avenue was put up for sale since the Clinic would be leaving this immediate area. It was ultimately sold to Mr. George Haupt in July of 1955 for $18,000. On July 15, 1954, Sidney Gassman, Ervin Thomas, William Cummings and their wives agreed to sell the house and property at West 312 Eighth Avenue to the Rockwood Holding Company for $60,000. Thomas and Gassman were the owners and operators of a fashionable men's clothing store in downtown Spokane and the owners of numerous other properties. The Holding Company paid $35,000 in earnest money and agreed to pay another $15,000 on completion of the transaction. $42,000 of this was in the form of a promissory note at 5% interest. The principal was to be paid off at $445 a month. The deal was contingent on partial release of the existing mortgage. The Holding Company also took an option on the Culmstock Lodge at South 711 Washington Street for $20,000.

The residence at West 312 Eighth Avenue had been called the Malcolm Brownlee mansion. Brownlee, had been a former Montana banker and an associate of copper king Marcus Daly. The turn of the century showplace had been built in the 1890's and at one time was one of the city's foremost social centers. More recently it had been used to house the overflow of tenants from the Culmstock Arms. The Culmstock Lodge was now needed by the Clinic to provide the parking space required by the city building code. When the architectural plans for the new building arrived in December, 1954, from Ellerbe and company there was great excitement for all concerned and the building committee was authorized to negotiate further financing.

A most important meeting of the partnership was held in March of 1955. Mrs. Robinson had contracted a serious illness and Dr. Robinson predicted her death within three months. In deference to her wishes he was anxious to keep working until her demise, agreeing to retire when this occurred on his drawing account alone. Some of the partners seriously questioned his physical ability to practice, however it was agreed to continue the existing arrangement for the time being. Partnership percentages as of that date were: Robinson—6.7%, Schlicke, Delaney, Copsey, Logan—12.7%, Wilder, Luther, Berghan—8.6%, Hempstead—6.9%, McIlvanie—2.9%. Although the outlook for Mrs. Robinson was grim, her death turned out to be not as imminent as feared, so in July of 1956 Dr. Robinson complied with the wishes of the partnership and retired on a drawing account of $900 a month.

In July of this year two new internists joined the staff. The first was Dr. David C. Bunch a graduate of the University of Mississippi and Louisiana State University. He interned at St. Joseph's Hospital in Kansas City, Missouri and had his graduate training along with some time on the staff at Henry Ford Hospital. He had served two tours of duty in the Navy before coming to Spokane and appeared on the scene here with a bristling crew cut. His subspecialty was in the field of allergy. His avocations were photography and later, mountain climbing. The second to arrive was Dr. Arthur B. Petersen who bore a striking resemblance to television celebrity, Ed Sullivan. He had attended Oregon State College and the University of Oregon Medical School and interned at Wesley Memorial Hospital in Chicago. He spent a year in medicine and pathology at the University of Oregon and then served four years as a fellow and staff member in medicine at the Mayo Clinic. Along the way he put in two years as a physician in the U.S. Air Force. Then in October the Clinic finally acquired the type of person it had been looking for to head up the Radiology Department, Dr. E. Finch Parsons, a tall, slender, gracious individual from Flushing, New York. He was a graduate of Yale who attended medical school at Columbia and interned at the Bryn Mawr Hospital in Pennsylvania. He spent some time at St. John's Episcopal Hospital in Brooklyn and at the U.S. Marine Hospital on Staten Island. Then after two years in the Air Force Medical Corps he took a three year residency in radiology at the Presbyterian Hospital in New York. Among his other accomplishments Finch later became a deacon and finally an ordained priest at the Episcopal Cathedral in Spokane.

Two other important steps were taken this year. At long last standard operating procedures were adopted for trip and vacation time and for retirement. It was decided that a retiring partner was to receive four months drawing account, four months of payments of the amount due him from his share of the distribution of profits, $200 for each year as a partner and the par value of his stock in the Rockwood Holding Company to be paid over a period of five years.

This was also a year of intense search for financing and for the best way of handling it from the Clinic's standpoint. An agreement was signed whereby all negotiations regarding the new building were to be conducted without liability to any retiring partner or to the estate of a deceased partner, the remaining partners to assume responsibility for any notes signed by the former. In these days all major loans required the signatures of all the doctors and their wives individually and it was not until 1958 that the Rockwood Holding Corporation was able to borrow on its own name. The term Corporation is here used correctly. The Internal Revenue Service had decided that there was a possibility that there might be small corporations which were not intrinsically dishonest or evil so on May 31, 1955, Articles of Incorporation of a new Rockwood Holding Corporation were filed and promptly certified by the Secretary of State of Washington.

All of the members of the Rockwood Holding Company, a co-partnership were involved. Under its license the Corporation was authorized to buy property, build, repair, borrow money, etc. in perpetuity. The by-laws provided for three directors and Dr. Logan was elected President, Luther Vice-President and Berghan Secretary-Treasurer with Jenkins as the Assistant Secretary-Treasurer. The Directors were authorized to issue 100,000 shares of common stock at $1.00 a share. The Rockwood Holding Company agreed to transfer to the Corporation all interest in the sale agreement with Gassman et al, subject to an existing obligation of $40,181. The eleven incorporators received certificates for 2000 shares of common stock in consideration of the transfer of the sales agreement to the Corporation. The president of the Corporation was directed to accept for the Corporation the sales agreement and the existing obligation. All of the assets, rights and obligations of the Company were ultimately transferred to the Corporation which was to be liable for all future payments on the existing contract on the property and for the purchase of supplies, equipment, furnishings, etc. No stock was to be disposed of without the approval of the remaining stockholders except that on the death or retirement of a stockholder his shares were to be sold back to the Corporation. Since the time when those changes were effected no further financial reorganization has been necessary and the Rockwood Holding Corporation continues up to the present to be the entity which holds all the fiscal assets, buildings, parking areas, and equipment which it leases to the Clinic and which collects rents from other lessees such as the pharmacy and the occupants of other buildings. Ellerbe and Company expressed a desire for a local architect to work with William Shannon, their staff architect, who had been assigned to the job here. Ellerbe was fortunate in securing the services of Mr. Victor Wulff who supervised the day to day progress of construction. With the experience of clinic requirements which Mr. Wulff gained on this project, he has been able to take care of all of the Clinic's architectural needs since the completion of the new building.

The desperate search for money continued. The Clinic's rent was raised from $2,000 to $3,000 a month. Then came the good news from the chairman of the building committee, Dr. Berghan, that he had received a verbal commitment from the Spokane and Eastern Branch of The Seattle First National Bank for $125,000 at 5% interest for interim financing. Then the Equitable Life Assurance Company of America approved a loan of $330,000 at 4¾% payable at $435 a month and secured by a mortgage on the property at West 312 Eighth Avenue and a note signed by the individual partners and their wives. $60,000 was borrowed from the Rockwood Clinic retainage fund at 4%. This was a fund maintained by withholding all of each partners net earnings for one year to serve as working capital. Mr. Platter who rented the space for his Pharmacy came up with $25,000 to be repaid over fifteen years at 5% interest. $20,000 was obtained from the Rocket Securities, an investment club whose members were for the most part Clinic doctors. Ellerbe and Company made a truly magnanimous move at this juncture by deferring $18,500 of their fee without interest, until the financial picture had cleared.

In March of 1956 the City Planning Commission approved the plans for the building and on the twenty-second of that month the bids for the building went out. The winning total was $600,000 with the Ruud Construction Company getting the general contract. This was a bit more than the Clinic had anticipated so Mr. Jenkins rushed down to the office of Mr. Edward A. Coon, executive vice-president of the Spokane and Eastern Branch. As Jenkins reports it, after hearing of the problem Mr. Coon said, "Well Arch, I don't think the Seattle First is going to let a little matter of $150,000 stand between these bids and a chance for Spokane to have an outstanding medical institution. Why don't you go on back and accept the bids?" Jenkins did and activity was soon under way at West 312 Eighth Avenue.

In the meantime a number of further real estate dealings had taken place. An easement for access was obtained from Gassman et al for $400. The property of a sweet little lady named Mae Heid who ran a tiny neighborhood grocery store at West 304 Seventh Avenue was bought for $25,000, $7500 down and $150 a month. Mrs. Heid was to continue residing there for $40 a month until the Clinic needed the premises. The purchase included the store-home, a full stock of groceries and a number of garages. It was planned to use the property for doctor parking and the dwelling as a home for the chief of maintenance. One of the great dates in the history of the Clinic was the day the groceries were distributed (equally?) among the members of the partnership. It was just like Christmas with each beneficiary waiting in childlike anticipation for his pile to see what goodies it contained. There was much argument and recrimination and charges of favoritism but everyone had a great time.

The Clinic took up its option on the Culmstock Lodge at South 711 Washington Street. The land on which it stood was needed for additional parking so the building was sold for $1500 with the stipulation that it be removed immediately. The purchasers were the members of a corporation hastily formed for the purpose, Mr. William Burch, an insurance executive, Dr. Berghan and Mr. George Nichols, the eminent real estate tycoon. The building was moved at great trouble and expense up the South Hill to a lot on Eleventh Avenue just off Rockwood Boulevard. It is still there but the Holding Corporation finally had to write the deal off as a bad debt based on the plea of poverty by the purchasers. The Clinic more than got even with one of these individuals, however, for the Foundation, to which the old Clinic building at West 66 Eighth had been reconveyed by the Rockwood Holding Corporation in 1951, sold this property to George Nichols for $95,000. Nichols then leased it to the Rockwood Clinic Partnership for $1500 a month until their new quarters were ready. He later sold it, along with the Robinson home and the adjacent Davenport-Porter mansion to an institution calling itself the Northwest Air College which purportedly had signed up 150 resident students whom it planned to train for jobs in the airline industry. This deal fell through when the operators decided that the old Clinic building was not suitable for administrative offices and classrooms and filed suit against Nichols and proposed to move out onto Inland Empire Way. He then converted the old Clinic building into a sort of motel and as this it continued until it was torn down, along with the Robinson home to make way for the new Sacred Heart Medical Center, the Sisters of Providence having in the meanwhile bought the properties.

Activity proceeded apace at West 312 Eighth. First the Brownlee mansion had to be torn down. Then came extensive excavation which would accommodate a foundation sturdy enough to support four more stories above the initial plant if they should ever be needed in the future. There was concern that the diggers might encounter lava deposits so common in the area which would have added greatly to the cost of this phase of the operation. Fortunately they did not but they did run into an underground river which to this day requires constant pumping to prevent a wash-out. The new building was to be of re-enforced concrete with brick facing, two stories high on Eighth Avenue, three stories on its north or downhill side with a full basement. In addition to examining and waiting rooms, business office, laboratory, a pediatric suite, a library, space was to be provided for both diagnostic and therapeutic radiology. While the building was still under construction, the Rockwood Holding Corporation leased the premises to the Rockwood Clinic for $6,000 a month subject to annual renegotiation. There was concern how all these new financial obligations and the payroll could be met. A special committee was appointed to study the problem. The recommendation with which they came up was a simple one. Everyone should buckle down and work even harder than he had been.

In 1956 the last payment of the donation to St. Luke's was made so the Foundation initiated the practice of awarding a $400 scholarship each year to several deserving students of medical technology at an Inland Empire college or university. In order to help assure an adequate supply of laboratory technologists in the community the recipients were required to practice in Spokane for a year after completing their internship or to repay the amount received to the Foundation. In July of this year two more internists were added to the staff. Dr. Ralph A. Kilby was a graduate of Williams College and the University of Buffalo Medical School. He interned at St. Barnabas Hospital in Newark, New Jersey. He spent a total of four years in the Navy and completed a fellowship in internal medicine at the Mayo Clinic. Ralph was an intellectual type and became president of the Spokane unit of the English Speaking Union. As Berghan had done before him he also played an active role in the local diabetes detection drives. Robert F. Kandel attended undergraduate and medical school at Duke University. He interned at the Aultman Hospital in Canton, Ohio, served as a naval officer for four years and then took a residency in medicine at the Henry Ford Hospital. He was the first Spokane physician elected to the American Rheumatism Association and later served as president of the Inland Empire Arthritis and Rheumatism Foundation. He was also very active in church work and taught classes in Sunday school.

With the dawn of 1957 Drs. Bunch, Petersen and Parsons were admitted to the partnership. Shortly after the first of the year the partners made their first tour of the new building with the architect. It was a thrilling experience but it was also apparent that the prime contractor was a long way from being able to meet his promised completion date of February 12. This was distressing for in addition to the payments of the rent and financing of the new building there was still the rent and other expenses of operating the old one, and the matter of keeping patients informed of plan changes. Some unbelievably torrid correspondence passed from Mr. Jenkins, normally a mild mannered gentleman, to Mr. Ruud. As it turned out the building was not ready for occupancy until May. When that time arrived all of the doctors had full appointment schedules in the old building on Friday, the third of May. On Saturday, May 4, with the help of the Lyon Van and Storage company and an enthusiastic crew of amateurs recruited from the Clinic's professional and lay staff the big move was accomplished in one day and at one third of the estimated cost. It was an exciting adventure kept afloat by several cases of beer and by Monday, May 6, everyone was back with a full schedule in the new building. As Arch Jenkins has said, "The staff was really overwhelmed finally to be in quarters built especially for themselves. Oh, there were bugs but nothing that couldn't be survived. There was a chart drop from the top to the bottom of the building with the only trouble being it was built to Mayo Clinic chart size. Ours being larger records, this vertical slide became the world's longest ash tray. The mechanical installations were placed in the north wing with the result that our later two story expansion caused the mechanical equipment to block out one of the world's most magnificent views. Obviously from a scenic standpoint, the mechanical wing should have been the west wing, then nothing would have been blocked. To those with an adventuresome spirit you can still see the view we blew if you will go to the top of the building through the elevator shaft, out the door, then up the ladder, and there it is in all its magnificence. Or have someone take you up some May 6. But all in all it's been a superior structure, especially when one compares it with other structures of equal age and usage....unfortunately Mount Spokane did not show up on a drawing board in St. Paul." Mr. Jenkins' allusion to a May 6 climb refers to a rite religiously carried out for many years by members of the building committee and certain selected guests.

One person to whom it would have meant so much never entered the new building. This was Dr. Robinson who had died at the age of fifty-nine while vacationing with Mrs. Robinson in Honolulu. "Thus ending," as Jenkins put it, "a truly amazing Spokane Saga." In 1951 Dr. Tobin had made a diagnosis of hypertension, coronary heart disease, angina pectoris, left bundle branch block and early calcareous aortic stenosis. In April, 1956, Dr. Robinson had an episode of acute chest pain and Dr. Delaney found him to be in acute left ventricular failure. A few months later his aortic murmur was getting louder and he developed mild dyspnea. Just before he left on what proved to be his last vacation he was found to be in better condition than he had been for a long time. At the time of his death February 5, 1957, he was found to have marked cardiac hypertrophy, severe calcific aortic stenosis, recent thrombosis of the anterior descending branch of the left coronary artery, congestive heart failure and pulmonary edema. The principle problem of his last two weeks of life, however, was progressive renal failure due to nephrosclerosis. How he carried on as well as he did as long as he did is unbelievable.

His estate was estimated at a little over $20,000, from the sale of his home next door to the old Clinic, a $10,000 group life insurance policy, his interest in his Hayden Lake home and some personal property. Whatever cash was left from the above after taxes was to be placed in a trust for Mrs. Robinson. Any stock in his name remaining in the Foundation, untouchable except for voting purposes, was willed to Schlicke.

Bill Robinson was a dreamer and at one time a hard worker. The institution which he had founded was on its way to becoming the realization of his fondest dream and with a degree of professional acceptance that his original enterprise was never able to attain. He never had a lot of money. He was more interested in growth, development and progress than in the accumulation of wealth. It would be incorrect to assume that he dug down in his jeans to build, and pay for a magnificent plant to hand over to his successors. He certainly got the show on the road by acquiring and arranging the financing of certain properties. He had been talented, industrious and a good doctor, whose reputation with the public was outstanding. Because of these attributes and the quality of his old hospital his credit rating was impeccable. So he was able to borrow most of the funds necessary to get things started and without which there would have been no Rockwood Clinic. Interestingly enough, the only doctor he was able personally to recruit after World War Two was Wendell Sharpe. It is unfortunate that for much of the time those of the present staff knew him, he was a very sick man. His robust appearance and bustling manner made this hard for them to realize. What they were most aware of was that he had left them a heritage of distrust and dislike in the professional community which it had taken them years to overcome. They were also disturbed because he never offered to take week-end or emergency call and after the first few years saw very few patients. This created a feeling of resentment which led to the harsh and uncompromising attitude toward any future member of the team who was unable to carry his full share of the work load, although this had long been held out as an inducement to prospective partners whereby attainment of parity by all was rendered equable by allowing older partners to slow down and have more time off. When it finally came to the point that there was no longer any continuity to the care Dr. Robinson was delivering and when even the quality of that care began to suffer there was no alternative to insisting on his retirement. There is no question that his successors owe him a debt of gratitude, for his enterprise, his ability, for a place to start practice, for a backlog of devoted patients. If Bill said you were all right just about anything you did was all right with them. On the other hand, it is important to remember that for a number of years he had a retirement program such as none of his sucessors could hope to attain.

At one of the last meetings held in the old building it was decided to reduce the number of years required for new partners to achieve equal participation in the Clinic earnings. The Spokane Society of Internal Medicine was making threats to withdraw from the Medical Service Bureau if it did not accept the internists' new fee schedule and the partnership agreed to do likewise if this occurred. In the meantime the partners sought legal advice regarding the problems of the radiology department with the Medical Service Bureau. The Bureau was still not paying the Clinic a cent for X-rays done on patients at the Clinic yet if such patients were sent to radiologists outside of the Clinic these physicians received full reimbursement. This was an affront to Dr. Parsons' ability and to the integrity of the staff besides representing unconscionable discrimination. Later in the year Dr. Parsons was sent to San Francisco for post graduate instruction in radiotherapy and it was voted to obtain appropriate radiotherapy equipment on the rental basis even though the Medical Service Bureau had assured the Clinic it would not be reimbursed for such treatments. An isotope laboratory was in operation by November under the direction of Dr. Parsons with the participation of the hematology department. During the year there had been frequent discussions as to whether to install a physical therapist in the building. Such discussions occurred periodically thereafter but nothing has come of them.

It was apparent to nearly everyone in 1957 that there would soon be a need for another general surgeon. Dr. Delaney objected, but as so often happened his views did not prevail. On the recommendation of Dr. John Waugh of the Mayo Clinic, who also happened to be Dr. Logan's brother-in-law, Dr. Edward V. Johnston came to visit the Clinic in July. He had been associated with a group in Waterloo, Iowa, and become increasingly unhappy there. He had attended Indiana University, obtained his M.D. degree at Northwestern University School of Medicine, and taken his internship at the Massachusetts General Hospital. He served two years in the Navy as a flight surgeon and then picked up a master's degree in anatomy at Northwestern while serving there as an anatomy instructor. There followed a fellowship in surgery at the Mayo Clinic 1950 to 1954, the last year as first assistant to Dr. Waugh. He liked what he saw when he visited Spokane, learned that the basic science examinations were being given in Seattle the next week, holed up in the Davenport Hotel for a couple of days to refresh his memory, took the examination, passed it without difficulty and accepted a job at the Rockwood Clinic, just like that!

Ed's first and most obvious interests besides surgery and his family when he came to Spokane were photography and putting together hi-fi equipment. It turned out that he was also an accomplished musician who played the saxophone and clarinet and had led an orchestra in high school and played with Will Bradley's band while in college. In Spokane he organized and arranged for a Doctors' band in which Arch Logan played the saxophone and a later arrival, Roy Zimmer, the trombone. He also made musical arrangements for high school choral groups and stage bands and sang in chorales and in the choir at St. John's Cathedral. Occasionally he would sit in with or "jam" with local musicians such as Arnie Caruthers and Don Eagle. One day he went to watch an unlimited hydroplane race, became fascinated and proceeded to build three consecutive top class limited hydroplanes which he raced in himself, attaining a high national rating. After a trip to Europe with his family he developed an interest in sculpture, tried a bust of his wife from local marble. Thereafter obtaining his marble from Carara, Italy he created a number of beautiful sculptures, one of which "Helen of Troy" won the best of show at a national exhibition of medical artists. An ardent gardener and weight lifter, his most recent interests have been ancient history and travel.

Drs. Kandel and Kilby were admitted to the partnership in 1958. Jenkins, who by now was proving invaluable, was to receive $10,000 a year, an extra allowance of $25 a month and an annual bonus equivalent to 2% of the Clinic profits. He had no voting rights, but his vacation time, sick leave and terminal gratuity were to be the same as those of the partners. A letter arrived from the Medical Service Bureau stating that henceforth the Clinic would receive full reimbursement for X-rays taken of Department of Labor and Industry patients, a miniscule portion of the Clinic's practice. It was, in any event, only a token concession so it was voted to retain legal counsel to look into the whole matter of Bureau discrimination against the radiology department. There was hope that relations between the Bureau and the Clinic might improve since the bureau trustees had filled two key positions with capable and reasonable people. Dr. Harold T. Pederson of the pre-World War Two Clinic became the medical director and E. Lee Clark the general manager.

A motion was passed to the effect that the practice of partners' children "soliciting" within the Clinic was frowned upon. This sounds like an eyebrow-raiser but it simply was designed to prevent cute little kids from cluttering up the place especially around the holidays selling trinkets, cookies and candy, albeit for worthwhile causes with Clinic personnel feeling obligated to purchase their wares. It was also decided that any sizable gifts to doctors were to go to the Foundation or the Partnership and not to individual partners. As the Christmas holiday approached, in an unprecedented burst of generosity the Clinic offered to make a $1,000 interest free loan available to new staff members if needed.

Earlier in the year the decision was reached not simply to duplicate the ortho-voltage radiotherapy equipment already available in Spokane, but instead to purchase a "cobalt bomb," a relatively new source of high voltage radiation for the treatment of malignant disease and the first such device in the Inland Empire. As it happened, Dr. Parsons attended the meeting at which this matter was discussed in his clerical garb. After the vote was taken and the project approved, Dr. Delaney turned to Dr. Parsons and said, "O.K., Finch, now you can turn your collar around." Finch was so delighted the partners were going to buy him this expensive toy that in a moment of misguided enthusiasm he assured them that his department would never require the services of another radiologist. In less than a year he was obliged to admit that his statement had been "a mistake." The Clinic not only relented by instituting a search for a second radiologist but bought a new additional diagnostic machine.

A part time dietitian was hired. After the untimely death of Paul Castoldi the legal work was divided between Nelson Repsold and Jack Dean who had served with Jenkins in the Army. The principle social occurrence of the year was the marriage of Dr. Robinson's widow, Mable, to an affable, well-to-do financier named Hugh McCall at Hayden Lake. In spite of her greivous illness of which Hugh was fully aware, Mable was still a beautiful woman and the union was a great source of happiness to them both and a particular comfort to Mable as her end approached.

In 1959 Dr. Johnston was admitted to the partnership and two more internists and a radiologist added to the staff. Dr. Thomas A. Marr was a graduate of the University of Minnesota Medical School. He interned and took a residency in internal medicine at King County Hospital and the Veterans Administration Hospital in Seattle. The years 1945 to 1946 he spent on duty in the Navy. He then had an eighteen month fellowship in nephrology with Dr. Belding Scribner at the University of Washington Medical School. Tom soon became the leading nephrologist in the area and organized the artificial kidney program at Sacred Heart Hospital which among other things, pioneered in the concept of home dialysis. Dr. William A. Dittman received his Bachelor of Arts and M.D. degrees from the University of Wisconsin. He had his internship and internal medicine residency at Salt Lake County General Hospital and the University of Utah, followed by a two year fellowship in hematology with Dr. M.M. Wintrobe in that city. Before coming to Spokane he spent a year in hematology at the Veterans Administration Hospital in Albuquerque, New Mexico. Bill also became an expert in the use of radio-active isotopes and is a dedicated teacher as well as practitioner. Dr. Robert M. Wilson, Jr. received his M.D. degree at the Medical College of Virginia in 1943 and in 1949 completed his internship and residency in radiology at the Medical College of Virginia Hospital with a two year interruption for service in the Army. He then worked as an associate radiologist on the Medical School staff and carried on a private practice until his arrival in Spokane. His energetic hobby was mountain climbing. His calm demeanor and gracious southern manner was a perfect balance for Dr. Parsons' chronic hyperkinetic state.

A new partnership agreement was signed with two significant changes. If a partner was unable to work for a period exceeding six months out of eighteen he was to receive no terminal gratuity in the event of his death or departure except the $200 per year of service allowance. Provision was made for sabbatical leave whereby partners would be entitled to twenty-two extra work days off after ten years in the partnership at the rate of ten days per year. Ten more days off were allowed after each additional five years, to be used within five years. Absence from the Clinic was never to be more than eight consecutive weeks and all such leaves were to be cleared with the Executive Committee.

The director of the laboratory, Miss Mary Ann Ripple, who had occupied this position since 1951 suffered a serious illness and was obliged to resign. A Ph.D. biochemist named Palmer Cox was hired to take her place. He arrived in January and in March submitted a letter indicating his desire to terminate in June. He was advised to be off the premises by March 31. A motion to install "piped music" throughout the Clinic was defeated. The request of a local attorney for Dr. Kandel to review all cases of patients with arthritis involved in litigation was denied.

Perhaps the most significant event affecting the Clinic in 1959 was the trial of the law-suit which Dr. S. Thatcher Hubbard, an anesthesiologist, had filed against the Medical Service Bureau alleging that it was a monopoly which restricted the practice of medicine in Spokane. This dragged on for over a month and Dr. Parsons and Mr. Jenkins were both subpoened to testify for Hubbard. He lost the case, Judge R.J. Ennis ruling that the Bureau was not a monopoly. However, the judge in his final review stated that the Medical Service Bureau should be enjoined from its discriminatory X-ray fee practices, such as not paying the Rockwood Clinic for X-rays of its own patients which were interpreted by Board Certified radiologists. The Clinic lost no time in writing to the Bureau to emphasize this point. Later Hubbard appealed to the Washington State Supreme Court which in 1962 upheld the verdict of the lower court and denied a motion for a new trial.

It became necessary during this year to ammend the Articles of Association of the William W. Robinson Medical Foundation, Inc. The Internal Revenue Service was making threats to remove its tax exempt status since it was not operating a hospital. It was pointed out to the I.R.S. that the post World War Two partnership was organized strictly as an out-patient clinic practice and had never entertained any plans of operating a hospital. Its sole sources of income were the payments of $150 a month from George Nichols and occasional voluntary contributions. The new Articles indicated that the Foundation was awarding scholarships, making charitable donations, subsidizing research. None of its earnings would ever enure to the benefit of any member, trustee or officer, nor would there ever be any sharing by them of any of the assets in the event of dissolution. It was authorized to hold real and personal property, dispose of same, borrow money and make investments. This document was filled with the Secretary of State of Washington and approved by the I.R.S. on August 26, 1959.

As the decade of the 1950's draws to a close it is of some interest to consider the changes which had taken place in the Clinic. The decade could hardly have begun more inauspiciously and yet with the passage of time things began looking better and better. Fifteen outstanding young physicians had been added to the staff, not counting temporary additions.

"The reputation of the group," to quote Jenkins, "was unassailable in Spokane, the Inland Empire and Western Canada. Half of the new patients came from out of the city and the doctor referrals were increasing, but it was the patients and friends of patients who really liked our mix as the best multispecialty group in the area and also as a place where they could find virtually total family care every day in the year." The most heartening thing for those who had been involved from the start was the gradual acceptance by the medical community which was taking place. A splendid new Clinic building had been erected. Debts were being paid. The business office had been reorganized under the guidance of the business manager with the assistance of a new accountant and was now operating according to sound business and management principles.

It is pleasant to scan some of the newspaper clippings from that era of growth and transition. In 1955 Schlicke was elected president of the Sacred Heart medical staff, a thing which would have been unthinkable just a few years earlier. He was also admitted to membership in several regional and national honorary surgical societies. Berghan was chairman of the Spokane County Medical Society diabetes committee. McIlvanie was being invited to give talks and was presenting the results of his researches at first locally, then regionally, nationally and finally internationally. He was also attracting substantial grants for his hematologic studies. Joe Delaney was president of the Northeast Branch of the Washington State Heart Association and widely quoted in the newspapers on his pronouncements. The next year he was president of the Spokane Society of Internal Medicine and then delegate to the governing body of the American Heart Association. In 1957, Schlicke was president of the Board of Incorporators of the Spokane and Inland Empire Blood Bank and the following year president elect of the Spokane Surgical Society. In 1958 he was appointed chairman of the Surgical Committee at Sacred Heart Hospital, a position he held until his retirement in 1975. Later in the year to everyone's amazement he was nominated for the presidency of the Spokane County Medical Society. He missed it by one vote but the ice was broken and since then three of the partners have attained this office. Chris Johnston began accumulating medals for his swimming prowess and Paul Schlicke's name was frequently on the Sport pages for his track activities.

12

HEALTH PROBLEMS

IT SOUNDED AS THOUGH things at last were really going the Clinic's way, and they were, but during this same decade of the fifties there occurred an incredible series of health problems, incredible because there were so many in such a small and basically healthy group of relatively young people. Harville's mild coronary at age forty-seven has already been mentioned. In 1951, Peggy Tobin (36) had a close brush with death. She was found by her obstetrician to have a placenta previa. When she was seven months pregnant she was admitted to Sacred Heart Hospital for close observation until she was near term. When this time arrived a low segment type of Cesarian section was carried out by Dr. Raymond E. Gillett. She proceeded to have a massive intrapartum hemorrhage due to a retained placenta accreta. The blood kept pouring out while consultation was obtained to justify a hysterectomy. Multiple transfusions were administered and Dr. Delbert Small did everything which a fine anesthesiologist could do to support her, but by the time the hysterectomy was performed she was nearly moribund. Happily she survived the operation, the bleeding was controlled, she had an uneventful convalescence and ended up with a fine little girl who is now a physician and married to an M.D. But it was a near thing.

In 1954 Dr. Robinson was finally able to convince his wife, now thirty-eight years old, to see a doctor after she had been having progressively heavier vaginal bleeding for a year. She was found to have an enormous, fungating, Stage III, grade IV squamous cell carcinoma of the cervix. She was sent to the Swedish Hospital Tumor Institute in Seattle where she received radium and X-ray therapy and then had her female organs removed by Dr. William Hutchinson. No residual tumor was seen by the pathologist but within three years she had developed pulmonary metastases. She did surprisingly well for a while but then required radiotherapy to her mediastinum and was started on chemotherapy. She carried on courageously until her death August 8, 1961.

In 1955, Joe Delaney (46) had a severe myocardial infarct. He was soon able to resume his practice and strenuous physical activity at his lake cottage, but elected to go off of the night and week-end call schedule. As time went on and he seemed quite vigorous, this decision aroused considerable resentment in an already sensitized group. He was virtually trouble free until 1966 when he had his second infarct and was put on anticoagulants. At the time of his third infarct two years later he went into congestive heart failure, but responded promptly to appropriate thereapy. He was again able to return to work and in spite of arrhythmias, mitral regurgitation, occasional pulmonary edema and gout he continued for another ten years, adamantly refusing to retire. Finally the volume and quality of his work had fallen off so badly that even those who had objected to his taking time off were now insisting that he retire in June, 1976. About three weeks later and just three months after the death of his wife from extensive carcinomatosis secondary to breast cancer, he had his final heart attack while driving his car east of town. His car went across two lanes of opposing traffic, fortunately without causing damage to anyone else, out into a field finally coming to a stop against a tree. By this time Joe was dead.

Also in 1955 Mary Luther (38) turned up with a hard solitary nodule in the right lobe of her thyroid gland. On removal it proved to be benign but its character had been worrisome.

Early in December, 1955, Nancy Bunch (34) who was six weeks overdue on her menses was found to have a huge left ovarian tumor which because of its character and rapid growth was highly suspicious of a malignancy. A pregnancy test was positive and on December 7, with considerable trepidation on the part of all concerned she was operated on. To everyone's joy she was found to have not one but two benign ovarian cysts. One was removed and the other aspirated and she went on to term and had a normal delivery of a fine little girl and three years later gave birth to a handsome boy.

In 1957, Tom Wilder (42) was hospitalized with chest pain. His electrocardiogram showed evidence of a coronary occlusion at least two months old, his present symptoms being due to coronary insufficiency. He took anticoagulants for a while but then felt so well he discontinued them. In 1960 he had some more angina and the anticoagulants were resumed. October 16, 1961, he and McCartan were out duck hunting. They separated for a brief time and McCartan heard three shots fired. When he returned to where he had left Tom he found him on the ground, dead of a heart attack. The sheriff's office notified the Clinic and Jenkins and Schlicke set out to notify Mrs. Wilder, speculating on the way how to break the news. On arrival they found her with a neighbor lady who had already heard the news on the radio and rushed over to be the first to tell Jean. It seems that the media monitor the police radio closely. Tom was a fine surgeon for whom his partners had a great affection. He was sorely missed. One cannot but wonder in this day of angiographic studies and aortocoronary bypass how things would have turned out if these modalities had been available when he first became aware of his heart problem.

Dr. Robinson's death in 1957 has already been recounted but he hardly fell into the category of the young and healthy ones. In that year, however, Art Petersen began to have a lot of abdominal pain and lost 20 pounds. It was found that he had developed a large gastric ulcer, possibly malignant. He had been dosing himself with a lot of antispasmodics and narcotics which led to a serious drug problem. He was sent back to the Mayo Clinic where Dr. James T. Priestley carried out a gastric resection for what proved to be a benign ulcer. In spite of this good news his problems continued and he became quite depressed. He finally agreed to go to Seattle for psychiatric treatment. The morning that he was to have his first appointment, September 5, 1958, he was found dead in his hotel room. He was thirty-seven years old. The King County Coroner called it an accidental death due to barbiturate poisoning.

Later that same month Dean Luther complained of headaches and visual disturbances which had been bothering him for two or three months, particularly the preceding two weeks. Copsey examined him and found that he had impaired visual fields (bitemporal hemianopsia). An X-ray of his skull showed a greatly enlarged sella turcica. He was forty-two years old and obviously had a rapidly growing pituitary tumor. He too was sent back to the Mayo Clinic where Dr. J. Grafton Love through a frontal approach removed a large pituitary adenoma which showed signs of recent hemorrhage. He made an uneventful recovery and has lived an active and useful life since.

Less than two months later Gayle Copsey, now forty-one, announced that he had been having some bleeding from his bowel. A sigmoidoscopic examination revealed the presence of an early malignant tumor. It just didn't seem possible. The endoscopist practically went into shock. A resection was successfully carried out. His convalescence, however, was not as rapid or smooth as one could have wished but the pathologist's report was encouraging and his long range outlook seemed good. In 1974 he developed some further polypoid lesions in other portions of his colon which had to be removed. Again the operation went well but this time he developed a severe delayed reaction to the anesthetic employed, ultimately making a good recovery.

Dave Bunch was also operated on in 1958, fortunately for nothing more serious than acute appendicitis.

In May of 1959 Sam McIlvanie (44) developed some enlarged lymph nodes in his neck. Biopsy revealed that he had Hodgkin's disease. He was sent back to the Sloan-Kettering Institute of the Memorial Hospital for Cancer and Allied Diseases in New York City, where he was treated with ultra high voltage radiotherapy and intravenous nitrogen mustard, obtaining an excellent response. When he returned to Spokane he was not only troubled by the usual post irradiation esophagitis but some long lasting and miserable symptoms of spinal cord and nerve root irritation. A few months after his return home he was hospitalized with acute abdominal pain. The fear was that he had developed abdominal extension of his Hodgkin's disease. However, after prolonged procrastination he was operated on and found to have plain old accute suppurative appendicitis. His convalescence from the appendectomy was uneventful.

The same month that Sam developed the lump in his neck Bob Berghan (39) came in with the same complaint. His lump proved to be a solitary nodule thought to be in the thyroid gland although there was some question of a parathyroid tumor since he had recently been troubled with kidney stones. At operation he was found to have a fetal adenoma of the thyroid and no abnormal parathyroid glands.

By the end of the decade this extraordinary succession of health woes had the partners wondering who had it in for them now. There have been health problems since but never in such a dramatic cluster.

13

PROPERTY ACQUISITIONS—MEDICAL SERVICE BUREAU—MEDICARE

At the first partnership meeting in 1960 it was voted to pursue the differences existing between the Clinic's X-ray department and the Medical Service Bureau including litigation if necessary to obtain reimbursement for diagnostic radiology. A few months later the Bureau announced that payments would be initiated but that the amount would be based on an averaging system which included all physician members of the Bureau. This was still not an equitable arrangement since there would be a tremendous difference between the number of X-rays ordered by a diagnostic clinic and say, a dermatologist. However, this ruling was not allowed to stand in the way of the purchase of additional much needed X-ray equipment which this time was financed through the Clinic rather than through the manufacturer. Another important decision stemmed from a victory by the devotees of constant cacophony and this was to install taped music in the Clinic waiting areas.

In August Dr. Kilby announced his intention to withdraw from the partnership, continuing on a monthly stipend until November. The remaining partners regretted his decision as they thought highly of him but realized that he was not happy in a nonacademic environment where his practice was mainly primary care rather than referral. He joined the Army Medical Corps for a while and then returned to a staff position at the Mayo Clinic. At about the same time Dr. Kandel was asked to resign, as Jenkins so charitably expressed it, "Based on a philosophy of patient care somewhat different from the norm and other considerations." It was agreed that he could continue as a hired doctor until the end of the year. Some, at least, of this time was spent by him abstracting information from his patients' charts. This led to a later amendment to the partnership agreement which stated unequivocally that medical records were the property of the partnership and that no one was to remove them or to extract information from them except in the performance of his duties as a member of the staff. Fortunately after being reminded of the two year restrictive clause to which he had agreed when he signed up, he decided to avoid a big hassle and returned to a staff position at the Henry Ford Hospital where he had trained.

This fall Schlicke was elected to the Board of Governors of the

American College of Surgeons. Not to be outdone, his son, Paul, became the state mile and cross country champion and a merit scholar finalist. Chris Johnston continued to accumulate swimming honors and his dad built and raced his first hydroplane. Joe Delaney addressed the Spokane Chamber of Commerce on "Socialized Medicine" and was a guest speaker at a dinner honoring the superintendent of schools. Elma Turner, who had worked in the prewar Clinic and then served as the head of the secretarial department since the opening of the post war Clinic retired after these many years of faithful service. Parsons and Bunch were elected stock holders in the Corporation, a new corporate agreement having been signed which proclaimed the eligibility of any new partner to become a stockholder after three and a half years in the Partnership. Drs. Parsons and Wilson had a brief try at furnishing fluoroscopic coverage and consultation to the Coulee Dam Hospital but this proved totally impractical and was soon abandoned.

Drs. Marr, Dittman and Wilson became partners January 1, 1961. At the first partnership meeting of the year a precedent making decision was reached when the partners allowed Bill Dittman to work half days at Sacred Heart Hospital. Many of the partners had traditionally devoted considerable time to teaching and preceptorship at the hospital, but Sacred Heart was looking for a hematologist and Bill wanted to have more of his practice hospital based, so it seemed that the proposed arrangement would strengthen the hematologic departments of both institutions and this proved to be the case. The Robinson Foundation approved a $2,000 grant to Sacred Heart Hospital for an artificial kidney (renal dialysis) machine. A motion to consider the request of two Spokane pediatricians to affiliate with the group was tabled by the partnership. The space which had been provided for a pediatric department in the new building was currently being utilized by the Insurance Department. Two stand-by pumps were installed in the basement as additional insurance against being washed away by the underground river. This stream unfortunately had only a nuisance value as its flow was not sufficiently predictable or dependable to permit its use for air conditioning. In March the first long range planning committee was established with Arch Logan as chairman. Marr, Schlicke and Jenkins were appointed to serve with him and were directed to meet at least quarterly. Dr. Copsey was appointed as chairman in charge of physician procurement. Dr. Victor E. Castleberry, a cardiologist, joined the Clinic staff in May. He was a graduate of Texas Technological College who earned his M.D. degree at the University of

Texas Medical Branch in Galveston. He served his internship and residency in internal medicine at the U.S. Public Health Hospital in Seattle, attaining the position of Senior Assistant Surgeon.

The Rocket Securities Investment Club was in the process of dissolving so the Holding Corporation picked up the note for the amount due. A new note was negotiated with the S. and E. Bank for the remaining $80,000 owed them, to be paid at $2,500 a month at 5½% interest. A $25,000 check was received from the Continental Assurance Company, the proceeds of a life insurance policy on Dr. Wilder. This was turned over to his estate. The stockholders of the Corporation also agreed to pay to his estate the book value of his 7,490 shares in the Corporation. Ten percent ($1640) was to be paid immediately and the remainder in nine equal annual installments. A contract was drawn up for the purchase of this stock from his widow and it was agreed that this should be the mechanism for buying back the stock of future retiring or deceased partners. This was truly a precedent making move, for prior to this time the stockholders had declined to attach any value to the shares until a sound financial base was assured. There was also talk that the Articles of Incorporation should be amended so as to make future investment in the Corporation by the partners optional. At this same meeting the first of numerous discussions took place concerning the possibility of forming a professional corporation for the practice of medicine, recent legislation having made this possible. A good deal of expert outside advice was sought but up to the present this has not seemed to be the direction in which the Partnership wished to move.

One Monday morning in June, 1961, Mr. MacEachern failed to appear for work. Little has been said about him for some time, mainly because there was little to say. His position had gradually become increasingly anomalous and a source of embarassment to Mr. Jenkins. There was no job description which could possibly be drawn up for what he was or was not doing. There was some cash missing the day he left but it was soon apparent that he had simply dipped into the till for the exact amount of his next pay check. He had apparently gone off on a self authorized and arranged sabbatical tour of the Northwest, finally turning up at his apartment some time later. The necessary funds were provided and Mac and his wife sent back to their ancestral home in Gloucester, Massachusettes.

This was the year that Dr. Delaney moderated a panel on coronary artery disease at the University of Washington. Ed Johnston won his first seven liter hydroplane race at the Pot Holes Inboard Regatta at Moses Lake. Paul Schlicke took five seconds off of the old record in the mile run at the State Track Meet at Pullman, turning in a time of 4:19:3. Sacred Heart Hospital built a $300,000 addition mainly for expanded administrative services. Molly Coburn, the Clinic's telephone operator was getting rave newspaper reviews for her performances with the Coeur d'Alene Civic Theater.

In 1962 Joe Delaney became president-elect of the Washington State Heart Association. Finch Parsons began his training for the Episcopal Ministry. The Executive Committee was expanded to four members and the term of service extended to two years. Honorariums received by members of the staff for guest appearances were to be donated to the Robinson Foundation.

There were three new additions to the staff. Dr. Roy W. Zimmer, a general surgeon arrived in July. He had attended undergraduate and medical school at the University of Wisconsin and interned at Fitzsimmons General Hospital in Denver. He served in the Air Force from 1953 to 1955 and then had a fellowship in surgery at the Mayo Clinic, and like Dr. Johnston before him he was first assistant to Dr. John Waugh. He had practiced for a year in Madison, Wisconsin before joining the Rockwood Clinic. In an organization which through the years boasted a number of enthusiastic golfers, Roy was the undisputed champ and even attained the ultimate glory of an authenticated hole in one. It goes without saying that he was also a first rate surgeon.

A few days after Dr. Zimmer's arrival, Dr. Rex T. Hoffmeister, a rheumatologist, joined the group. He had had his undergraduate and graduate work at the University of Nebraska, and interned at the Nebraska Methodist Hospital. He spent two years in the Army in Germany and then had a three year fellowship in internal medicine at the Mayo Clinic. The third new arrival came in November. This was Dr. John H. Phillips, a hematologist. He received his B.A. at Cornell University in 1950 and his M.D. at Columbia in 1954. He interned at King County Hospital in Seattle, had a residency in internal medicine at Roosevelt Hospital in New York City and at the New Hampshire Veterans Hospital. He then served a fellowship in clinical hematology at the University of Washington.

In the financial department the Gassman et al note was paid up. A promissory note was negotiated with the S.&E. Bank for $40,749 to be paid at $1,000 a month at 5½% interest. The Holding Corporation was authorized to offer Mrs. Gianetsas $50,000 for a handsome old home which had been converted into apartments at South 703 Washington Street. Amazingly it was obtained for $49,000! Presumably since she did not live there she was more amenable than when the Clinic attempted to purchase her home on Eighth Avenue. A down payment of $10,000 was made and a mortgage for $39,000 signed with the stipulation that the building was not to be demolished until $5,000 more had been paid. George Mitchell, who had replaced Charles Tilson several years earlier as head technician in the X-ray Department operated it as an apartment house until the space was needed for additional parking. Three months later, in early 1963, the Corporation was finally able to secure the lot at West 311 Seventh Avenue with its ramshackle buildings which was grandly called the "C.H. and Myrtle Isherwood property" but referred to by the partners as the "Chicken Coops." An attempt had been made to acquire this property in 1956 but the difference between the $10,000 the Corporation offered and the $50,000 the owner wanted could not be resolved. The $35,000 finally paid seemed exorbitant but it made it possible to get rid of a real eyesore and ultimately to provide more parking space.

1962 was the year Bob Berghan was president of the Spokane Society of Internal Medicine and that Ed Johnston won his greatest hydroplane victories, beating the legendary Bill Muncey in the seven liter class race at Newman Lake.

At the beginning of 1963 Dr. Victor Castleberry became a partner. There were now sixteen partners and three salaried physicians. As the Clinic had grown so had the amount of paper work. Maintaining good medical records has always been an essential part of good medical practice. Filling out insurance forms, although a boring chore, is a requisite if patients are to collect from their carriers for their medical bills. Prompt attention to correspondence with patients and referring physicians is not only common courtesy but most important from a public relations standpoint. What should be done about the occasional staff member who was habitually in arrears? It was finally decided that such delinquents would lose one half day of vacation time for each week they were behind. One exemplary member of the staff was appointed to monitor this activity.

Joe Delaney was elected president of the Washington State Heart Association and was off on a round of speeches. His wife, Eleanor, who had recently undergone a radical mastectomy for a most unfavorable tumor, was elected president of the Spokane Women's Symphony

Association. Ed Johnston was ranked second in the national point standings in seven liter hydroplane racing. At the annual meeting of the stockholders of the Rockwood Holding Corporation there was a good deal of discussion regarding the properties which had been acquired, how the payment of debts was progressing and what future capital commitments might be in the offing. A most important decision was made at this meeting whereby management was directed to begin accumulating funds toward the retirement of stock of retiring or deceased stockholders. The setting aside of funds for this purpose has continued to the present.

There were further meetings and correspondence between the partners and the Medical Service Bureau regarding the inequity of the averaging scheme in connection with reimbursement for diagnostic radiologic procedures. A detailed cost analysis of the recently instituted radiotherapy program was carried out. At the annual dinner meeting of the Medical Service Bureau the names of three individuals were selected for submission to the trustees as candidates to fill a vacancy on the Board of Incorporators. Amazingly one of them was a Clinic partner. He received excellent support from the membership but was not chosen by the Board. The time was not yet ripe, but it seemed that it was not beyond the realm of possibility that some day the Clinic would have a representative on the Board which would be the best step imaginable toward helping to solve the problems which persisted between the Clinic and the Bureau.

In September the Washington State Medical Association met in Spokane. Schlicke served as program chairman. The theme was Space Age Medicine and numerous international celebrities in this field participated in the program. An innovation was the presentation of the region's first closed circuit medical television program. A live showing of an open heart operation from Sacred Heart Hospital was broadcast to the meeting site. The mechanics of setting up this pioneer project proved as interesting as the show itself.

In 1964 Drs. Phillips, Hoffmeister and Zimmer were elected to partnership. Electrophoresis equipment was procured for the laboratory, a new $15,548 cobalt source for radiotherapy and laminography unit for diagnostic radiology. A cytologist was employed to screen Papanicolaou smears, final readings being by a pathologist. The partnership decided that henceforth contributions to hospitals, charities and public service projects, excepting those handled by the Foundation would be on an individual basis. At about this time it was decided that the name of the Dr. William W. Robinson Foundation, Inc. should be changed back to the

Rockwood Clinic Medical Foundation, Inc. Contributions were beginning to come in in increasing amounts and frequency and it was thought better to identify this charitable corporation with the name of the institution rather than that of an individual. This was not done out of any lack of appreciation for what Dr. Robinson had accomplished but was felt to be more appropriate in the light of present circumstances as a means of implementing its charitable objectives and attracting donations and bequests. The final approval from the Secretary of State of Washington was not obtained until three years later.

Much of what occurred this year can be gleaned from newspaper clippings. Copsey became president of the Washington State Society of Internal Medicine and Schlicke, who was the current president of the North Pacific Surgical Association was chosen as president-elect of the Washington State Medical Association. Miss Regina Zappone, who had served long and faithfully as supervisor of receptionists left to get married. She was replaced by Mrs. William (Betty) Barton. Paul Schlicke who was now captain of the Stanford University track team ran a 4:02 minute mile. Ed Johnston won the Region Ten high point hydroplane racing trophy in the seven liter class.

The year was catastrophic for our accountant, Carl Nicholson. His wife, Audry, was killed in a head on automobile collision just south of Spokane. Less than a year later Carl was sentenced to serve six months in the Federal Penitentiary on McNeil Island for failing to file income tax returns for the previous six years. It was difficult for everyone to understand how such a thing could happen, particularly in the case of a C.P.A. Fortunately there was never any suspicion of peculation as far as his dealings with the Clinic were concerned and the Clinic will always stand in his debt since it was through him that it acquired one of the greatest assets it ever had in the person of its business manager, Arch Jenkins. After these events Mr. Donald Schoedel, C.P.A. took over the accounting chores and has continued to perform those functions up to the present.

In 1965 for the first time serious attention was directed to a comparison of the production figures of the individual partners. The results of this financial survey were reviewed by the Executive Committee but otherwise were kept "top secret." There was not felt to be enough disparity to warrant considering any change in the equal sharing system. In fact the only change which resulted was a reduction in the time required to attain equal partnership from five years to four years after the preliminary probation period of eighteen to twenty-four months.

Anxiety began to be expressed regarding the ethics of the pharmacy lease. The pharmacy was on the premises as a convenience to patients and at no time were they under any obligation to patronize it. However, there did seem to be grounds for a conflict of interest in an arrangement where the rent was contingent on the pharmacy's income. Three years later when the current lease expired a new lease was signed under which the pharmacy paid a fixed monthly income based on the footage of the space occupied.

An autoanalyzer was purchased for $12,000 for the laboratory and a new diagnostic X-ray unit with an image intensifier was leased for the radiology department, which also acquired an additional supply of radium. In a moment of extraordinary largess the partners decided that anyone having sufficient enterprise to write a magazine article or a book or had the necessary talent to earn prize money or an honorarium should be allowed to keep any money he received. Grants and bequests would still go to the Foundation, but those so designated could be earmarked for research by a specific partner. All other money earned outside of the Clinic such as for consultations, legal testimony, etc. was to go into the Clinic hopper.

An unsuccessful attempt was made to acquire the miniscule backyard of the Oxford apartments at Seventh and Bernard to improve access to the new lower parking lot, but it was not long before rumors began to circulate that the entire property might soon be available for $75,000. In the meanwhile acoustical tile was installed in the corridors of the Clinic building and new carpeting in the reception areas.

Individual accomplishments this year included: the selection of Tom Marr as director of the Inland Empire Artificial Kidney Center at Sacred Heart Hospital; Gayle Copsey was president of the Spokane Society of Internal Medicine; Sam McIlvanie who had also held this position, was elected president of the Medical Staff at Sacred Heart Hospital. Rex Hoffmeister became Medical Committee Chairman of the Inland Empire Arthritis Foundation. Articles appeared inthe papers about Finch Parsons and his cobalt bomb. Chris Johnston won a National Amateur Union junior swimming title.

With the advent of 1966 the Clinic was again suffering growing pains. A new building committee was appointed with Dave Bunch as chairman. Discussions were initiated with Victor Wulff and with the bankers regarding an addition to the building. Victor Wulff had acquired sufficient knowledge of the refinements of clinic construction as a result of his role vis-a-vis Ellerbe so that no out of town consultants would be needed this time. It was disappointing to learn that because of a recent minor earthquake in Seattle which had shaken the cornices off of a few old buildings that changes in the building code had been made which would prevent the addition of more than two stories plus a penthouse library and meeting room. This meant that any further expansion in the future would have to be lateral rather than vertical.

In March there was further correspondence with the Medical Service Bureau regarding full payment for diagnostic radiology. Two months later the Bureau agreed to average the Clinic's reimbursement for X-rays with those ordered by other internists. This was comparable to what was done for other services rendered and far more equable than any previous arrangement. In September the Bureau even agreed to pay $17 per treatment for radiotherapy.

For some time there had been some agitation to close the Clinic on either Wednesday or Saturday. Rather than doing this the partners decided to give all of the doctors an extra half day off, thus putting everyone on a four and a half day work week. One half hour less was to be taken off for lunch.

In July Dr. George M. Pavey, an internist and gastroenterologist joined the staff. He was a graduate of South Eastern Missouri State College and obtained his M.D. degree from the University of Missouri. He interned and had a three year residency in internal medicine at the University of Missouri's Kansas City General Hospital. Between 1953 and 1955 he had served in the Army. He had no sooner arrived than he wanted the Clinic to buy him a gastroscope and a laparoscope. The present generation of fiberoptic gastroscopes was a far cry from the old one Sharpe had ordered. With Pavey's enthusiasm and skill the new instrument was soon put to extensive use and a whole new vista was opened up in diagnostic gastroenterology. Regarding the laparoscope there was considerable foot-dragging as this was an instrument which the surgeons felt should preferably be utilized by a surgeon. Once he had his new toys and a little league baseball team to coach, Pavey caused no further trouble, but others were soon clamoring for their share. A treadmill was purchased for the cardiologists. The equipment needed by the radiologists to do mammographic studies was leased rather than bought because of the rapid technological modifications being effected.

On July 1, 1966, the implementation of Public Law 89-93, the Medicare Act, began. At the Rockwood Clinic the transition took place surprisingly smoothly due to the careful planning of the business office. The Clinic followed the advice of the American Medical Association and billed all patients directly, taking assignments only when the other option would create hardship. Another reason that there was so little confusion connected with the change was that it was administered locally by the Medical Service Bureau. In spite of the differences which through the years had existed between the Bureau and the Clinic there was no question in anyone's mind that the Bureau was the best agency to serve as the intermediary with the Department of Health, Education and Welfare (H.E.W.).

One of Schlicke's first big assignments when he became president of the WSMA was to accompany two representatives of the Washington Physicians' Service back to the headquarters of HEW at Bethesda, Maryland to see whether approval could be obtained for the Medical Service Bureaus to serve as the medicare intermediaries in the state of Washington. The meeting was to take place early on a Monday morning in December, 1965. Since the meeting was of such importance, flying so uncertain at that time of year and the prediction being for dense fog in Spokane, Schlicke raced over to Seattle in his car on Saturday evening, parking it at Sea-Tac Airport. To the surprise of all of the passengers on the night plane for the East which he took, the first stop was in Spokane where the plane was grounded for mechanical problems. He spent the night at the Spokane Airport while efforts were being made to get him to his destination. Early the next morning he departed and three airlines later was on the last plane to get into Washington Friendship Airport in a pea soup fog. Bright and early Monday morning the three Washington representatives, now accompanied by a two man Idaho delegation on a similar mission headed for HEW headquarters. The HEW official presiding at the meeting interrupted the Washington presentation, saying, "You don't need to tell us about your program. We are thoroughly familiar with it and have used it as one of our models." This was nice to hear and a tribute to the pioneer efforts of the people who had set up the Bureau in response to the Great Depression of 1929. The Washington representatives were virtually assured that their mission had been successful as it later proved to have been. The Idaho people were not so fortunate.

There was much other excitement during these years that President Lyndon B. Johnson was trying to establish his "Great Society." There were countless talks to County Medical Societies and other groups attempting to explain the legislation being enacted by Congress which affected health care and to ease the transition into Medicare and Medicaid. There was the "Partnership in Health" legislation which inaugurated comprehensive health planning. It was a great idea, but in its original form it was doomed to failure from the start for those involved in implementing it spent much of their time raising matching funds to support the program and were not provided with "teeth" to enforce compliance with their recommendations. Locally this involved service on Governor Daniel J. Evans' Washington State Comprehensive Health Planning Council. Then there was the Regional Medical Program (RMP) in response to the DeBakey Commission report on the conquest of heart disease, cancer and stroke. The more objectionable features of the report, such as sending patients with these conditions to a handful of super-centers, were eliminated in the legislation which passed. Public Law 89-239, garnered considerable support from the medical profession as a means of establishing good programs of continuing medical education and improving the availability and quality of care to victims of the three big killers. There were consultations with the University of Washington Medical School and with Governor Evans and service with the Washington-Alaska RMP Advisory Board. The program itself ultimately perished for lack of funding.

There were two memorable White House Conferences. One of these even included cocktails and dinner at the White House. Mr. Johnson was convalescing from a cholecystectomy so Vice President and Mrs. Hubert Humphrey served as hosts. It was obvious that the support of the medical profession was needed to make any of these programs work and the Administration was out to get it. One heard Secretary of HEW, John Gardner, emphasize that good health was a basic human right. One became familiar with the term, the "disadvantaged." One was exposed to what then seemed like wild notions about compulsory continuing education and relicensing, controls, surveillance, monitoring, utilization review, all of which are now with us. Former HEW Secretary Marion Folsom advocated the elimination of fee for service solo practice, a philosophy exemplified today in the government push for Health Maintainance Organizations.

In general, relations with officialdom at a state level were good. The governor formed a personal medical advisory board which met with him frequently in Olympia. He appointed several physicians to a committee which was to study the facilities and operations of the legislature. However, when his Vocational Rehabilitation staff members began demanding that physicians sign a pledge that they would treat the "clients" of this department "without discrimination as to race, color, or national origin" a vigorous protest was raised that this was a reflection on the integrity and humanity of the medical profession.

There was one tragedy this year, PFC Will P. Barton, the son of our reception supervisor, Betty Barton, was killed in combat in Viet Nam. He had just shipped out from San Diego the week before with the 101st Airborn Division and was out on his first patrol. There was little that anyone could say that was meaningful by way of condolence. There was also a near-miss. The fly-wheel of Ed Johnston's hydroplane, *Annie's Dodge*, disintegrated during a race and stove a big hole in the bottom of his boat. Fortunately he had built this boat with a "cab-over" design in which the driver was seated in front of the motor or the Clinic could have been looking for another surgeon. Instead, he and Bill Dittman were elected to serve as delegates to the Washington State Medical Association.

The year 1967 was marked by prolonged hassles with the state Department of Public Assistance regarding reimbursement. Relationships deteriorated to the point that there was even a motion made at a partnership meeting that the Clinic no longer offer services to welfare patients but this was overwhelmingly defeated.

During this year the Spokane Eye Clinic and the Spokane Optical Company were involved in litigation. The Optical Company maintained a shop in the Eye Clinic building. This was a great convenience to patients and they were not restricted from going elsewhere to get their glasses if they chose. The allegation was that it was unethical to refer patients to a shop in which the doctor had an interest and that "kick-backs" were occurring. The implications to the Rockwood Clinic or any other clinic which had a pharmacy on its premises or maintained a laboratory or X-ray department were obvious if the plaintiffs prevailed. The case ultimately went to the Washington State Supreme Court and the Rockwood Clinic through its attorney Jack Dean, filed a brief of amicus curiae. Fortunately for the concept of clinic practice the Court ruled in favor of the defendants as long as statements of ownership were made public and certain other conditions met.

Jenkins was instructed to conduct a study of the Clinic's total organization, viz. the Partnership, Corporation and Foundation and in view of the recent Keogh legislation passed by Congress, to investigate pension programs. This he did with the help of a Seattle attorney, Jack Lycette, who was an expert in such matters. His advice, which coincided with the feelings of the partners, was that the Rockwood Clinic should continue to conduct its medical practice as a partnership rather than as a corporation and that a Keogh type retirement plan should be adopted. In June the adoption of such a plan was unanimously endorsed by the partners with financing to be carried out through the Fidelity Capital Fund. By January, 1968, the plan was fully operational with the blessings of the Internal Revenue Service forthcoming in March.

In 1967 amended by-laws of the Rockwood Clinic Medical Foundation were adopted. Qualifications for membership were provided: Rockwood Clinic partners, retired partners, Clinic Business Manager. Membership would be revoked if a member moved away, resigned, was expelled or died! Seven to fifteen trustees were to be elected and officers chosen. Officers and trustees were to be indemnified by the corporation in the event of legal action against them in connection with the pursuit of their duties.

Early this year the Building Committee was authorized to proceed with Victor Wulff as architect to draw up plans for expansion of the physical plant and parking areas. In October the architect's preliminary plans were presented. At this point in time the Clinic was desperately seeking additional physicians for the staff but the United States was still involved in the ill fated war in Viet Nam and good, well trained, young doctors were in short supply. Accordingly at the November meeting of the Partnership it was voted to defer detailed architectural planning until efforts at recruiting had met with greater success.

In the meantime Sacred Heart Hospital had been informed by the Fire Marshal that a significant portion of its patient care area was a fire trap and was proceeding with plans for an entirely new structure, a good portion of which would be on the old Rockwood Clinic site at West 66 Eighth Avenue. These plans included expansion and modernization of the radiotherapy department including the installation of a linear accelerator. It seemed foolish for the Rockwood Clinic to be offering these same expensive services just a block and a half away. Preliminary conversations between the Sisters and the Clinic were initiated and at Dr. Parsons' urging, interest was expressed in our performing the radiotherapy for the Hospital. Two years later a contract to effect this was signed.

Arrangements were made with Jennings Bacon who was providing after hours telephone call service to make a radio call service available to the doctors on call. A formal cardio-pulmonary resuscitation standard operating procedure was established and the necessary equipment kept readily accessible whenever the Clinic was open.

A momentous event occurred this year when after all the years of struggle and argument Ed Johnston was elected president of the Medical Service Bureau. This was the organization of the purveyors of service and not the policy making body but it was recognition and a step in an important direction. He was also serving as a delegate to the Washington State Medical Association. Schlicke was elected president of the Mayo Clinic Alumni Association.

On the first of January, 1968, George Pavey became a member of the partnership. A short while later Dr. Thomas H. Reed, a dermatologist, agreed to join the staff when he completed his three year fellowship in dermatology in July. He was a graduate of Whitman College in Walla Walla and received his M.D. degree at the University of Washington Medical School. He interned at Fitzsimmons General Hospital and then spent a year in internal medicine before starting his fellowship at the University of Washington. He had served as an enlisted man and later as an officer in the Army before starting medical school. Tom was the first true liberal to join the staff and his forthright expression of his views was at times quite disturbing to some of the more conservative members but in general had a stimulating effect and provided some much needed political balance. He became president of the Spokane Citizens for Abortion Reform, chairman of the Board of Planned Parenthood of Spokane, a participant in various liberal and environmental causes and was in much demand as a speaker.

Later in the year the Clinic finally acquired its first ophthalmologist. Dr. Jonathan A. Holloway. The closest the clinic had come before was eleven years earlier when it negotiated with a mountain of a man named Truman Davis. He was a delightful and well trained individual but his price tag was a bit high for that time. As it turned out his size and strength stood him in good stead after his visit to Spokane for when he headed east he was mauled by a bear in Glacier National Park. Jon Holloway was a graduate of Oberlin College and the University of Washington Medical School and interned at San Francisco City and County Hospital. He spent two years in the Air Force as a flight Surgeon and after a year at the University of Pennsylvania Hospital he had a residency in ophthalmology at the Wills Eye Hospital in Philadelphia. Before coming to the Clinic he had been associated with one of Spokane's most distinguished ophthalmologists, Dr. Andrew DeRoetth until his retirement. Jon was a man of many talents who used to come roaring up to the Clinic on his motorcycle. His interests included back packing, sailing and photography and he was a trustee and at one time vice president of the Spokane Symphony Society. Later he followed in Finch Parson's footsteps and became a deacon at St. John's Episcopal Cathedral. One of his greatest contributions to the medical community was his assumption of the editorship of the Spokane County Medical Bulletin which he changed from a shabby throw-away to an attractive, readable and informative journal.

At about the time Jon joined the Clinic negotiations were under way with another ophthalmologist, Dr. Alan Mackay, a graduate of the University of Vermont Medical School where his father was the Professor of Surgery. He joined the staff in 1969. The addition of these two specialists required rather extensive architectural changes in the building to accommodate their specific needs which resulted in the elimination of the old library-cum-lunch room. They also required an incredible amount of complex and expensive equipment. The Clinic reimbursed Dr. Holloway for the equipment he brought with him, while new equipment was purchased for Dr. Mackay with the understanding that he would buy it back if he didn't join the partnership.

Dr. Richard R. Stacey, an internist and rheumatologist, was also signed up to start when he finished his fellowship at the Mayo Clinic early in 1969. He was a graduate of Dartmouth and of Tufts Medical School. After interning at Philadelphia Presbyterian Hospital he served two years with the Peace Corps in Turkey. Dick already had some roots in Spokane where his sister was married to an eminent newspaper publisher. Moreover his wife, Connie, was a Spokane girl. He had also spent some time working in the office of Dr. William Myhre, a scholarly and prominent local internist.

With these prospective additions to the staff and more in the offing the Building Committee was instructed to resume activity. Furthermore the stockholders of the Holding Corporation at their May meeting voted to purchase The Oxford Apartments at Seventh Avenue and Bernard Street for $90,000 and the old Texaco Service Station at the northeast corner of Seventh Avenue and Washington Street for $45,000, the latter to be used for record storage and additional parking. $63,000 was borrowed from the Clinic by the Holding Corporation to make the down payments and to pave the south end of the Oxford lot. This loan was to be repaid at $451 a month at 6% interest. Because of the general depletion of the Holding Corporation bank balance the Clinic rent was raised to $7,000 a month. At their September meeting the stockholders voted to proceed with the addition of two stories and a penthouse to the Clinic building. The S. and E. Bank agreed to do the financing so Victor Wulff was authorized to proceed with detailed architectural plans. $15,000 worth of automated equipment was acquired for the laboratory. While all this was going on, just up the street, on September 12, 1968, ground was broken for the new $35,000,000 Sacred Heart Medical Center.

Upon the recommendation of the internists the partners voted to close down the Clinic on Saturday afternoons. The advent of Medicare had aggravated the paperwork problem so the Executive Committee was authorized to do whatever was necessary including withholding of pay of delinquent doctors in order to keep things up to date. A committee was appointed to look into Dr. Delaney's request to work less than full time. Upon its recommendation new disability rules were laid down. No partner was to reduce his work load unless disabled as determined by a Clinic Disability Board and approved by the Partnership. Any partner with permanent partial disability would be required to retire and become a salaried physician under a negotiated contract. An exception was made in Delaney's case allowing him to remain a partner until the mandatory retirement age of sixty-five, but he and any future partners exempted from being on the "on-call schedule" were to forfeit the equivalent of five percent of a senior partner's income for this indulgence.

In December Arch Logan became president of the Spokane County Medical Society, the first of the Clinic group to attain this honor. It would be difficult for those who did not experience the early troubled years to realize what this manifestation of acceptance by the medical community meant to those who lived through them. Earlier in the year one of the local newspapers had sought to do a "profile" on one of the partners but this was declined. Dr. Logan's accomplishment meant more than pages of newsprint. Tom Reed received an appointment as Clinical Instructor in Dermatology at the University of Washington and later was advanced to Clinical Assistant Professor.

In 1969, John Platter who had been operating the pharmacy since its inception merged with another pharmacist, Norman Scheer who continued the operation after John's retirement in 1976. It was always a pleasure as well as being a great convenience having such fine people as tenants, providing service to the Clinic patients and the community at large.

Victor Wulff had the plans for the addition to the building completed on schedule and bidding was opened on April fourth. To everyone's dismay, since only $600,000 had been budgeted, the lowest bid was $720,000 with Max Kuhne and Co. as the general contractor. However there was unanimous agreement by the partnership to proceed with full financing even though it might result in some loss of personal income. The S. & E. Bank granted a ten year mortgage loan for $718,000 at 3¾% to be repaid at $5,894 a month. The Clinic's rent was increased to $13,000 a month for the first year and $10,000 a month thereafter and this lease, the pharmacy lease and the mortgages on four parcels of land assigned as collateral. As Jenkins has pointed out, this was the first time in its history that the Corporation was able to borrow on its own name, "no cosigners, no wives, no Clinic." The Clinic, out of the retained earnings fund, did pick up all the outstanding loans on the previous building project and the Corporation agreed to pay back this $200,000 at 4¾% interest at $1,141 a month. Dr. Bunch, the chairman of the Building Committee urged all "to be calm and considerate of each other and of the employees" during the building phase.

The Clinic at this time was requested by the director of the Washington-Alaska Regional Medical Program to offer short term refresher preceptorships to general practitioners. After much debate it was decided to comply with this request but nothing ever came of it. In view of some recent malpractice litigation which was settled out of court, Mr. Jenkins reminded the partners of the importance of obtaining "informed consent" for all surgical or hazardous or investigative medical procedures or treatments. The approval of the Research Committee was to be obtained before the use of any experimental drugs. In September an SMA 12/60 autoanalyzer was leased for the laboratory. For the first time individual partners' production figures were revealed at a regular meeting. Occasionally a motion was passed or a rule made which deserved preserving for posterity, e.g. "Although it is *absolutely forbidden* to take charts from the building, anyone doing so....is urgently requested to notify the chart room personnel in writing of the whereabouts of the record."

At year's end Holloway, Mackay and Stacey were elected to partnership. Dr. Carroll S. Simpson, a cardiologist whom Berghan had discovered when he accompanied a patient to Cleveland was offered a position on the staff. Simpson was a graduate of Kansas University and the University of Missouri Medical School. He had spent five years at the Cleveland Clinic as a resident in internal medicine and a fellow in cardiology. He would bring to the Rockwood Clinic new skills in cardiac catheterization and angiography when he joined the staff, which he did in March of 1970.

Winding up the decade there were now twenty-four partners counting the three who had just been voted in. Valuable adjacent property had been acquired for parking and possible future expansion. The disasters of the previous decade had been survived and the Clinic had emerged as a strong institution widely recognized as an outstanding diagnostic and treatment center. An excellent relationship had been developed with Sacred Heart Hospital and rapport with the medical community was steadily improving in spite of the inevitable feeling of competition and occasional resentment which exists between any medical group and individual practitioners. One reason the Clinic was running so smoothly and prospering aside from the abilities of its professional staff and the qualities of its business manager was that it had been able to attract a corps of key employees of great loyalty and ability. Ray Lawson who brooked no interference in the manner in which he ran central supply had been with the post war Clinic almost from its start. Others who came in the fifties included Rosy Hebert who had started as a telephone operator, later filling in wherever she was needed and finally becoming an incomparable credit manager; Irene Qualtieri who took Elma Turner's place as head of the secretarial department, prompt and neat in her work, respected and liked by her "girls," always obliging; Annie Luders, head nurse for many years, hard working, capable, always cheerful and an inveterate practical joker; a series of tremendous scrub nurses like Helen Emery, Donna Dyer and Paula McPherson; Betty Barton who replaced Regina Zappone as supervisor of receptionists and served with competence, tact, and dedication; George Mitchell, chief technician in radiology and landlord extraordinary; heads of the laboratory like Mary Ann Ripple and later Robbi Gandini until Vic Castleberry married her and deprived the Clinic of her services.

14

THE COMPUTER AGE—SACRED HEART MEDICAL CENTER

1970 BEGAN WITH THE PURCHASE of a defibrillator to augment the Clinic's cardio-pulmonary resuscitation capability. Dr. Paul A. Beale, a diagnostic radiologist who had his undergraduate, graduate and post graduate training at Ohio State University was signed on to start work in July. He had also spent two years as a general medical officer at Fairchild Air Force Base. $25,000 worth of remodeling was carried out in the X-ray department to make way for a fourth diagnostic unit which was leased as soon as the space became available. Dr. John W. Harrison, an internist and rheumatologist who had been practicing in Spokane since 1960 as a member of a now defunct medical partnership expressed a desire to affiliate with the Clinic. He was well known and highly respected by the internists and had a large following of loyal patients. He had graduated from Washington and Jefferson College and the University of Pennsylvania Medical School. His post graduate training was at Lankenau Hospital and Bunts Institute of the Cleveland Clinic. He was a past president of the Northwest Rheumatology Society. However, he had some serious health problems so he was offered a contract as a salaried physician. This was not to his liking so it was agreed that he should start on a salary in March and then become elegible for consideration for partnership at the end of the year. He was elected to partnership at that time and proved to be a hard working, popular and valuable member of the organization until he was forced by progressive deterioration of his health to resign as a partner in 1976 and finally in 1977 to retire completely from the practice of medicine.

On March 9, five months after the estimated completion date the new addition to the building was ready for occupancy. (frontis) Only the new third floor was initially used for doctor's offices and examining rooms. The fourth floor was left unfinished until needed but in the meanwhile was used for the storage of records, for the secretarial pool and for the telephone switchboard. The pent-house proved to be an unexpected delight. For the first time the doctors enjoyed the luxury of a spacious meeting room and library, nicely furnished and decorated, and a place where they could eat their sandwiches, relax and admire the beautiful view. However the activities and acquisitions of the past year had exhausted the resources of the Holding Corporation so it was a time to pause and take stock. The April meeting of the Partnership was largely devoted to a consideration of what the future of the Rockwood Clinic might be in view of the many influences, activities, events and eventualities facing American Medicine. At least as Jenkins said "We were the proud possessors of a plant worth well over two million invested, with debts scarcely half of that. Outside the mortgage, the Rockwood Clinic was beholden to no one. The active medical staff owned it all....The whole lay-out stood and stands as a living tribute to the determination and dedication of all Rockwood Clinic doctors/partners, and" he added, "some may say fairly good administration."

A new planning committee was formed called the "Where Do We Go? Committee" (WDWG). The previous one had become inactive. This one met regularly and enthusiastically for a few years but regrettably in the long run its members tended to lose interest because of the low acceptance rate of their suggestions by the partners. Finch Parsons was authorized to take additional post graduate training in radiotherapy to prepare him to take over the direction of the Sacred Heart Medical Center radiotherapy department the following year. Arch Jenkins was directed to take the steps necessary to move the business office into computerized data processing. Sadly, after ardently supporting the American Association of Medical Clinics for many years the Clinic was becoming disenchanted for a number of reasons not the least of which was concern over that organization's increasing administrative costs and bureaucratic nature. A little over two years later the Clinic formally withdrew.

Ed Johnston was elected secretary-treasurer of the Medical Service Corporation, the governing body of the Bureau. When one thinks of all the unpleasant conflicts and confrontations of past years it was hard to believe that there was at last a direct voice to the policy making level of the Medical Service Bureau. This same year Ed was elected president of the Spokane Surgical Society. Arch Logan was chosen as a trustee of the Washington State Medical Association and Tom Marr was appointed to the Regional Advisory Committee of the Washington-Alaska Regional Medical Program. Governor Evans appointed Dick Stacey to the Washington State Comprehensive Health Planning Advisory Council. The Spokane County Medical Society instituted a new award, "Physician of the Year" and Schlicke was proud to be its first recipient. In August the Copsey's daughter, Cristine, had married James C. Mareau with the Rev. Dr. E. Finch Parsons performing the ceremony.

With the beginning of 1971 Simpson and Harrison were admitted to the partnership. Since the Clinic was going out of the radiotherapy business it was voted to donate the cobalt unit to Sacred Heart Medical Center, with them to pick up the tab for dismantling, moving and service as well as the remaining contract on the radioactive source. The benefits of having Ed Johnston on the Board of Incorporators of the M.S.B. were soon apparent when for the first time reimbursement for interdepartmental referrals within the Clinic and for urinalyses was allowed. Simpson was instructed to initiate a search for another cardiologist and Parsons to seek another radiotherapist to help him run the department at Sacred Heart. A new $36,000 table was leased for the X-ray department. The "Where Do We Go" Committee carried out a detailed study regarding future professional staffing of the Clinic and reported back to the partnership. The concensus seemed to be that for the foreseeable future its destiny would be chiefly as a medical-surgical clinic and that there was no point in trying to branch out into a Noah's Ark type clinic with two representatives in each and every subspecialty.

After years of discussions, tabling and rejection of motions the Partnership finally decided to close the Clinic entirely all day Saturday starting in June, 1972. The main rational for keeping it open had been to make it available to people who worked on week days. However, with each passing year fewer of them chose to avail themselves of this opportunity. Although the week day census continued to rise, the number of patients appearing on Saturday declined. Moreover it was becoming increasingly difficult to keep good non-medical help on Saturdays. The change resulted in very few complaints from patients. Paul Beale was elected to partnership and the time required to attain senior partnership and equal profit sharing was reduced to three years following the probation period for him and all future additions. The Clinic rent was raised $1,000 a month to prepare for the financing of the demolition of the apartment building at South 703 Washington Street and conversion of the property into a parking lot, which it was estimated would cost in the vicinity of $40,000. When this actually took place a year later, the cost of the demolition, paving, landscaping and lighting came to $59,500 but the Clinic was able to finance it without outside borrowing.

And then personal tragedy struck again, this time, for the first time to one of the younger generation. One evening in late June, 1971, Gayle Copsey's son, Steve, was driving home from Coeur d'Alene Lake with his date when a drunken driver came onto the wrong side of the freeway from an off ramp. Steve swerved to avoid a head on collision and his car overturned and rolled down an embankment. His young lady passenger received only minor injuries but Steve suffered massive intra-cranial trauma and never regained consciousness. He was taken to the intensive care ward at the old Sacred Heart Hospital. There was no evidence of anything localized like a blood clot which could be benefitted by an operation—simply diffuse brain damage. Because of his robust constitution and the absence of other injuries he lingered on for the better part of a week before expiring. This was a terrible ordeal for the rest of his family including his newly married sister who had come up from her home in Portland. It was also a great source of sorrow to the older partners who had known this fine young man since infancy and to their children who had grown up with him.

In October at the time of the meeting of the Holding Corporation it was voted that in the future interest would be paid on notes executed by the Corporation for the purchase of stock from retiring or deceased members at the same rate as an S. & E. Bank certificate of deposit.

Without a doubt the most exciting event of 1971 was the dedication of the new Sacred Heart Medical Center on October 29. Schlicke was privileged to be asked to preside over this momentous function. One of the principle addresses, "The Development of A Medical Center" was delivered by Dick McCartan who was the current President of the Medical Staff. Other participants included the Very Reverend Richard Coombs—Invocation, Bishop Bernard Topel—Blessing, Sister Ethel Richardson—Welcome, Sister Alice Hutubise, Asst. Superior General, Sisters of Providence-Greetings, Sister Margaret Vincent, President of the Catholic Hospital Association—Dedication Address, James McGoldrick, President of the Spokane Chamber of Commerce and Mayor Pro Tem Del Jones—Observations, Gus Bouten, Contractor and Tibor Freesz, Architect—presentation of keys, Sister Peter Claver—acceptance of keys. How fortunate the Clinic was to have this magnificent new structure with all the latest equipment just a block and a half away, where its patients were always welcome and assured of good care.

Ed Johnston who was currently serving as president of the Spokane Surgical Society was chosen president-elect of the Spokane County Medical Society and Dick Stacey as a trustee. Ed was also made president of the Medical Service Corporation this year. Schlicke was elected president of the Western Surgical Association at its annual meeting in Portland. He was also the first resident of the Inland Empire ever to be elected to membership in the prestigious American Surgical Association in which he was privileged to serve as second vice-president a few years later.

Paul Beale signed the partnership agreement and became the twenty-seventh partner with the advent of 1972. Dr. Donald A. Schmutz, radiotherapist signed up in January and started work in July. Don was a Cornell Medical School graduate who interned at St. Luke's Hospital in New York. After two years in the Army he served a residency in therapeutic radiology at the Geisinger Medical Center in Danville, Pennsylvania and was an associate on the staff there for three years before coming to Spokane. Attorney Karl Krogue was engaged to carry out a study of the feasibility of incorporation instead of partnership. At a later meeting attended by C.P.A. Don Schoedel he presented the pros and cons as they would affect the Clinic. Little enthusiasm was expressed by the Partnership for a change. A movement to abolish the retainage principle was spear-headed by Alan Mackay. Under the existing arrangement all partners had left one year's income with the Clinic as working capital. This had greatly expedited the financing of past major building projects and acquisitions. In January the partners voted to retain the principle. Nonetheless alternate plans kept surfacing and in September it was voted to abolish the present retainage system and substitute a specific dollar amount in the vicinity of $25,000 which a new partner would have five years to put in. The main benefit would be the increased amount a new partner would receive during his early years.

Strange real estate ideas began to float around about this time. One was to sell the Clinic building and move into one of the post World War Two wings of the Sacred Heart complex. A real estate firm offered to buy the Clinic building and rent it back to the Clinic. Neither option aroused any interest. Instead, a $15,000 renovation of the laboratory was agreed upon. Incidentally the laboratory was inspected by the State Department of Health in connection with certification under Medicare and received high marks.

The "Where Do We Go" Committee met with Roger Shannon the brilliant radiotherapist and computer expert from Holy Family Hospital to discuss multiphasic screening and the application of computer technology to medical practice. Less than a month later the word was out that his grants had expired and that the Hospital's computer program was in dire financial straits. The committee decided to investigate no further for the time being.

In May the Clinic received word that henceforth the M.S.B. was prepared to provide full reimbursement for diagnostic radiology. It certainly didn't hurt to have Ed Johnston in the top position on the governing body of the Bureau but there had also been a gradual transition in the character of this board as new members replaced the old toward a more liberal and less prejudiced stance. How much better it was, although it took much longer and required infinite patience, that the long standing inequities could be gradually eliminated in this fashion rather than by litigation.

Changes were voted in the "sabbatical" rules. Each partner would be eligible for an extra month off after fifteen years of service and two extra weeks off each year after twenty years of service, although time off was never to exceed eight weeks in a single year. Dean Luther who had been doing a superb job with his hip replacement operations was sent back to the Mayo Clinic to familiarize himself with the technique of total knee replacement. On his return, the first patient upon whom he performed this procedure developed a fever and leukocytosis several days after the operation. Dean was sure she had developed a wound infection which in a procedure of this type is a catastrophe of the first magnitude. Fortunately, before he seriously considered taking his own life, an astute surgeon came to his rescue by discovering that the cause of the febrile reaction was a silent but acutely inflamed gallbladder.

In November, Dr. Lowell T. Mouser, a cardiologist accepted an invitation to join the staff as of the first of the new year. Tom was a graduate of the West Virginia School of Medicine. He completed his residency in internal medicine and cardiology at that institution and then served as the director of the cardiac catheterization laboratory. He had previously been in Spokane between 1967 and 1970 at the Veterans Administration Hospital. Before going into medicine he served four years in the U.S. Air Force, part of the time as a Russian language interpreter. He currently has an appointment as Clinical Assistant Professor in the Division of Cardiology at the University of Washington.

At the December meeting of the County Medical Society Ed Johnston was installed as president and Arch Logan received the Physician of the Year Award. The Clinic also received the good news that the Internal Revenue Service which had just completed an audit on the Clinic's property depreciation schedules had no fault to find or reason to change the Clinic's tax status.

There was one bad scare in 1972. On November 8, Roy Zimmer, one of the Clinic's more vigorous members and now aged forty-four was hospitalized because he had been having some exertional substernal chest pain for the past month. Angiography revealed some rather alarming changes in his coronary arteries so a triple aortocoronary bypass was carried out by Dr. Ralph Berg. His convalescence was fortunately uneventful and he has continued to carry a full load of his customary high quality surgery and to maintain his status as a top flight golfer.

Early in 1973 a search began for a surgeon with extensive experience in vascular work and for a second orthopedist. Partners' production figures were again displayed with the usual surprising findings. Numerous suggestions regarding distribution of profits were brought up but it was voted to wait until the Clinic had been "on computer" for at least a year before considering any change. The volume of radiotherapy was steadily increasing but the department was still a long way from breaking even financially. Under Carroll Simpson's guidance the "Code 5" operation (cardio-pulmonary resuscitation) was brought up to date and formal instruction instituted for the doctors and other personnel. Because of his increasing cardiac problems it was decided to work out a new contract for Joe Delaney in order to give him more time off, but workless days were to be payless days.

In general it was an unusually calm and peaceful year except for two events. In September Alan Mackay resigned from the partnership saying that he wanted more control over his own practice. A partnership is not unlike a marriage in some respects; there has to be a certain amount of give and take and each partner must make some concessions for the good of the union if it is to survive. There are some individuals who are happiest working as part of a team and willing to sacrifice certain prerogatives for what they regard as the advantages of this type of practice. Alan was a fine ophthalmologist and a likeable person but from the first he objected to many of the rules, procedures and even forms which the partnership had found essential for smooth and efficient functioning. Numerous changes had been made to mollify him, most notably the elimination of the rêtainage principle. He was unalterably opposed to the restrictive clause in the partnership agreement whereby a partner severing relations with the group was prohibited from practicing within Spokane County for the ensuing two years. When he left he wished this waived in his case. The Clinic declined to do this and after considerable discussion between the lawyers of both parties Alan proceeded to spend the first two years in pathology at the Deaconess Hospital before reopening an office for the solo practice of ophthalmology. Although there had long been a certain amount of friction between the two ophthalmologists when the actual parting occurred it turned out to be on a more amicable basis than one would have expected. It was just that Alan should never have joined a group. Happily, he remains a friend.

Shortly after Alan's departure Sam McIlvanie, now fifty-eight years old who seemed to have gained a total victory over his Hodgkin's disease, was hospitalized because of chest pain of one week's duration. He was found to have a severe occlusion of his right coronary artery and was operated on immediately, a double aortocoronary bypass being performed. His recovery was rapid and it was not long before he was back at work seeing patients and tending his sheep.

The preceding year the fire marshal and the building inspector had become quite upset about the condition of the Oxford apartments. The options were to make some extensive renovations in order to comply with the fire safety code or to raze the building. For a number of reasons including tax benefits the former course seemed preferable at this time and was pursued at a cost of approximately $15,000. Even so, because of the benefits from the new addition, remodeling and the donation of the cobalt unit, the Corporation ended up this year in the black to the tune of $8,327 in contrast to a deficit of $15,000 the preceding year. The interest income which the Foundation had been receiving from the sale of the old properties to George Nichols ended when Sacred Heart Medical Center took them over and paid a lump sum. However more and larger contributions continued to trickle in and by 1973 its assets amounted to $4,692 in cash and $17,524 in a Security investment fund. The Foundation continued to award four scholarships a year and make generous contributions to a Washington State University Foundation. It also helped to underwrite some of the more expensive research projects being carried out by members of the professional staff.

On the political front Arch Logan was chosen as president-elect of the Washington State Medical Association. Also in 1973 a momentous change took place at Sacred Heart Medical Center. Just two years after moving into the new Medical Center the Sisters of Providence decided to expand their hospital governing body. Prior to this the Board of Directors had consisted of a group of about five local Sisters. It was determined that additional nuns from outside of the hospital religious community would be eligible to serve as would certain selected lay persons. The bylaws provided that no less than a majority plus one other member of the Board should always be Sisters of Providence. Members were to be elected annually by the St. Ignatius Provincial Council whose approval would also be required for any changes in the by-laws, real estate dealings or incurrence of any long term indebtedness. Initially in addition to several Sisters two business men, a psychologist and one physician were added to the Board. Moreover the President of the Medical staff was to be an ex-officio member of the Board without vote. It must have been a difficult adjustment for the Sisters suddenly to begin sharing decisions and prerogatives with people from outside of their Order and yet it provided them with a closer tie-in with the community at large, gave them access to a broader base of expertise and was in keeping with the new spirit of ecumenicism. Schlicke regarded himself as singularly fortunate in being chosen as one of the additions to the Board. He also considered it as an opportunity in a small way to make some recompense to the Sisters for their kindness and service to him, his colleagues, the medical community and above all to their patients.

In January, 1974, Mouser and Schmutz signed the partnership agreement. The Science and Research Committee expressed concern regarding the Clinic's vulnerability because of the use of certain hazardous and unapproved drugs, particularly in the hematology-oncology department. More stringent rules and monitoring were instituted and the importance of informed consent, protocols and detailed records was emphasized.

In February, to everyone's regret, Annie Luders, who had worked for the Clinic so hard and well for over twenty years as head nurse, retired and a party as given in her honor in the penthouse. This same month Dr. Warren R. Peters was signed up as the fourth surgeon, to start work in September. Warren was a graduate of Walla Walla College and Loma Linda Medical School. He had his internship and residency at the Virginia Mason Clinic in Seattle and came to the Rockwood Clinic very highly recommended by his former preceptors and skilled in vascular surgery. A few months after his arrival one of his most difficult operations turned out to be on Arch Jenkins, who had developed a huge aneurysm of his abdominal aorta. Arch was now sixty years old and quite a bit overweight but he had the necessary confidence in the new young surgeon and Warren had the necessary courage and ability so everything went nicely when the aneurysm was resected and a bifurcation graft inserted. Warren was a devout Seventh Day Adventist and soon became deeply involved in schools, health clinics and other church projects.

With the arrival of Peters, Schlicke volunteered to cut back on his operative schedule from three to two days a week and to restrict himself to three major cases on each of these days. Although he had a year to go before mandatory retirement it seemed prudent to start this gradual transition while he still had some patient drawing power in the hope of attaining a fairly equal distribution of the work load in the surgical department. In March, Joe Delaney having reached the age of sixty-five retired as a partner but signed a contract to continue as a salaried physician.

One of the fringe benefits of the computer program was that this arcane apparatus was now storing diagnoses for each patient visit. This made it necessary for each doctor to enter a diagnosis on the sheet provided for the purpose each time he saw a patient. Aside from making diagnoses available for research and review this also made it a great deal easier for a doctor to pick up a chart and tell at a glance the salient features of a patient's health history.

The "Where Do We Go" Committee after its study of staff needs recommended that a search be instituted for a neurologist, a pulmonary specialist, an oto-rhino-laryngologist, a cardiologist and some others. Arch Jenkins practically went into shock. The need for periodic infusions of new blood he regarded as a manifestation of the "grow or perish" syndrome. It was probably one of the only things on which he and the doctors were ever in disagreement. On the part of the doctors it was not so much an insatiable craving for growth but with the rapid advances taking place in medical science, a necessary means of keeping up on what was being taught in medical schools and training programs and of acquiring new techniques, ideas and view-points. It was a matter of not getting into a rut in a non-academic environment and not just "bigger is better."

Aside from the perpetual problem of keeping the doctors abreast of their paper work there was the matter of a chronic shortage of space for carrying out patient examinations. The doctors' offices had been designed not only as home bases but as examining rooms, yet some of the staff seemed to deliberately clutter up their offices with old letters, insurance forms, books, journals and other impedimenta so that there was no room into which a patient could be squeezed. Countless rules, regulations and solutions were repeatedly invoked but the problem persists.

Ed Johnston who had the biggest physical frame in the Clinic wanted the book shelves in the penthouse raised to a more convenient height. He was advised that if he found the level of the shelves a problem he should take off some weight. But it wasn't all rebuffs for Ed this year. He was re-elected president of the Board of Trustees of the Medical Service Corporation and later in the year was elected president of the Western

Conference of Prepaid Medical Service Plans. In May the Spokane County Medical Society honored him by naming him Physician of the Year. This was the third time in its short history that the award had gone to a Rockwood Clinic partner. In September Arch Logan moved up to the presidency of the Washington State Medical Association and Carroll Simpson became president of the Northeastern Chapter of the Washington State Heart Association. Meanwhile Carroll was busy giving talks to the Spokane County Bar Association and other groups. Schlicke who for a number a years had been a member of the University of Washington Medical School faculty was named Clinical Professor of Surgery.

The summer of 1974 was an exciting one because the only World's Fair of the decade which was to be held in the United States was staged in Spokane. Although the citizens of Spokane had voted down several bond issues for a fair, when EXPO '74 actually took place their enthusiasm knew no bounds. It was not just watching fireworks from the penthouse or marvelous entertainment and exhibits and lots of fun but it changed the whole nature of the riverfront and downtown area, gave the city many lasting improvements such as a beautiful park, an opera house, convention center and others, but most of all it breathed new life into the business community and instilled a degree of civic pride into the citizenry such as had never existed before. There was no longer any room in Spokane for "urban blight."

In December the Clinic won the Ockert vs. Rockwood Clinic and Finch Parsons malpractice case. This was the first time a case involving the post war Clinic had ever gotten as far as a jury. One previous suit had been dismissed by the judge and three other claims had been settled out of court. In the litigious climate of the sixties and seventies this was not a bad record considering the number and variety of patients seen during this time.

On December 20, a special meeting of the partnership was held at which Bob Berghan, who had recently divorced his wife and remarried, announced that he would be resigning early in 1975. For reasons best known to himself he had signed on with the Hospital Corporation of America to serve as an internist at the new King Faisal Specialty Hospital in Ryadh, Saudi Arabia. When he arrived there early the next year one of his first patients was a man who had been shot. Berghan worked long and hard to resuscitate him even after it was apparent that the patient was dead. Perhaps he was inspired to continue his efforts by the presence of a number of tommy-gun toting guards. It was not until he finally gave up that he learned that his patient was King Faisal who had been assassinated by his nephew.

By the close of this year the Foundation had received over $6,000 in grants and contributions. The Holding Corporation had spent approximately $15,000 remodeling the laboratory and the X-ray department.

15

THE OLD GUARD BEGINS TO FADE AWAY

AT THE OUTSET OF 1975 Bonnie Highfield, who had been running the laboratory since Robbi Gandini's departure announced that she would be retiring at the end of the year. Berghan's departure on the other hand was with only two months advance notice. Bob had been a loyal and popular member of the staff, except for his tour of duty in the Navy, since 1948. He was a first rate internist and endocrinologist with a large following of patients and his ingratiating manner had won him a host of friends in the community. However his sudden and unexpected withdrawal left the Clinic in the lurch without an endocrinologist, without provision for the coverage of his patients, and as it turned out, with a disastrous malpractice suit involving one of his patients, just after the partners had been congratulating themselves on their previous experience in this arena. The case was scheduled to go to trial at about the time that Berghan left.

The law-suit involved the 41-year-old wife of a friend of Berghan's, Attorney Lee Driscoll. She died suddenly and unexpectedly leaving her eight children motherless. It was alleged that the interaction of an anti-depressant drug called parnate with an over-the-counter diet pill "X-1" was responsible for her demise. The defendants were Robert Berghan who had prescribed parnate, his wife, Smith, Klein and French Laboratories, the manufacturer of parnate, and Porter and Dietsch, Inc., the manufacturers of a diet pill she had also been taking. Arch Jenkins describes one session in the Clinic library at which there were nine attorneys present, representing the plaintiff and the various defendants. Frank Johnson, the counsel for the Aetna Casualty Company, which furnished the Clinic's malpractice coverage, ultimately advised settlement, being of the opinion that there had been inadequate attention to "informed consent" and other matters and in consideration of the potential impact of the bereaved husband and the motherless children on a jury. The award agreed upon involved $60,000 from Aetna, $60,000 from Smith, Klein and French and $10,000 from Porter and Dietsch. This was by far the largest settlement in which the Clinic was ever involved and as is so often the case, many physicians felt that the case should have been allowed to go to trial and been vigorously defended. The partnership minutes tell that on the eve of his departure Berghan was presented with an expensive pair of binoculars as a "going away" present and as a "token of apparently unanimous esteem."

The "Where Do We Go" Committee recommended employing a pulmonary specialist, another general internist, a third radiologist, an orthopedist and an endocrinologist. It also recommended remodeling the second floor to accommodate some of these people. Holloway's quarters in the old library would be moved to the area which had been designed as the pediatric wing and which more recently had been under consideration for housing a nose and throat specialist. This and other changes would involve extensive renovation but could be accomplished for about $50,000 whereas finishing in the fourth floor would run in the vicinity of $175,000.

In March Schlicke retired as a partner but the partnership graciously agreed to have him continue as a full time employed surgeon subject to annual renewal of his contract. In May an elegant party was held at the Spokane Club for old timers Delaney and Schlicke. It was a great gathering much enjoyed by all and particularly appreciated by the honored guests. Delaney was presented with a gas grill and a $200 gift certificate for meat to cook on it. Schlicke and his wife were awarded a trip to Mexico with two weeks off with pay in order to enjoy it.

In May Jenkins announced that he planned the nurture and training of one Ralph Gamon as a possible replacement for himself when he retired. Ralph was born and raised in Spokane. He was a graduate of Lewis and Clark High School and earned a B.A. degree in Business Administration at Washington State University in 1967. He had held numerous managerial positions and for the past five years had worked for the Data Processing Services, Inc. of Spokane as a systems analyst and supervisor of the programming department. The "Where Do We Go" Committee was instructed to review Joe Delaney's practice with the objective of recommending his future role with the Clinic. The committee came to the conclusion that both the quality and volume of his work had fallen off to such an extent that he should be asked to retire completely in the fall. The partnership concurred but changed the date to July 1, 1976, in order to allow him time to adjust and for the Clinic to find a replacement. This was a difficult decision in view of his past outstanding service and the fact that by this time his wife Eleanor was suffering from widespread metastases from her breast cancer. She had had her second breast removed and was receiving both radio and chemotherapy and Joe wanted to keep busy. A year later she had developed paraplegia from spinal metastases and on April 24, 1976, she expired. Because of the emotional trauma involved in getting Joe to quit work a motion was made at the July meeting of the Partnership that there be no further employment at the Rockwood Clinic for partners after their retirement at sixty-five. Someone pointed out that this might work an undue hardship on those who for financial reasons still needed to work and that if this was to be considered the restrictive clause should be dropped at an earlier age in order to give a partner time to make other arrangements. The motion about rehiring was tabled but it was later voted to eliminate the restrictive clause when a partner reached age sixty-two.

In June it was decided to create the position of medical coordinator. The person occupying this position essentially would be an administrative chairman of the Department of Internal Medicine. He would have no duties in connection with the surgeons except regarding paper work, medical records, etc. Dick Stacey was elected to fill this position which would also involve ex-officio membership on the executive and "W.D.W.G." committees. Tom Marr who now had an appointment as Clinical Assistant Professor of Medicine at the University of Washington took over as medical director of the laboratory, a position which Berghan had held for a number of years. In July Guillermo Rubio, a Henry Ford Hospital trained endocrinologist signed on to start work in December. He had had his undergraduate education at the Instituto Patria in Mexico City, and received his M.D. degree from the Universidad Nacional Autonoma de Mexico.

Dr. Carl G. Oeljen, an orthopaedist started work in August. He was a graduate of the University of Minnesota Medical School who had done his post graduate work at the University of Wisconsin. He had also had a year of orthopedics in the Army in Viet Nam. He brought with him special expertise in the dissolution of protruded intervertebral discs by the injection of papain, but shortly after his arrival the use of proteolytic agents for this purpose was banned by the Food and Drug Administration. Come September our long sought and much needed pulmonary specialist, Lang Dayton, arrived. He had received his training at the University of West Virginia School of Medicine. Unfortunately things never worked out. He was a highly intelligent young man but there seemed to be constant problems of communication with both the staff and with his patients and he was asked to resign in February, 1976, which he did and left for a hospital position in California.

Upon the recommendation of the "W.D.W.G." committee the partners adopted a resolution that anyone planning to move away or to retire before the mandatory retirement age should be required to resign immediately. However, any partner or hired doctor was to feel free to meet with the "W.D.W.G." committee to discuss any problems or plans without prejudice and in strict confidence. It was also decided that the chairman of the Executive Committee should automatically become an ex-officio member of the "W.D.W.G." committee.

One of the great blessings of modern science from which the clinic benefited during this year was the replacement of the comfortable old telephone system by a shiny new "Dimension" installation. This sophisticated device seemed to have capabilities far beyond the needs (or understanding) of the average citizen and reduced to a minimum the contact with the Clinic's friendly switchboard operators. One of its more unpleasant features was that it would snarl at any user who absent-mindedly dawdled while dialing instead of paying strict attention to business. Worst of all it seemed miles beyond capacities of some of the less malleable doctors.

Ed Johnston was elected secretary-treasurer of the Washington State Medical Association. Because of his political aptitudes it was hoped this would lead into the presidency. However because of his disapproval of some of the Association's fiscal policies and some personality differences Ed chose not to serve further at the end of one year's term. With the leadership he had displayed in other positions of this type which he had held this was a disappointment to those who had urged him to take the position in the first place and a loss to the Association.

The year 1976 was a time of extensive changes in the staff and of visits by a large number of candidates. Warren Peters became a partner and a new partnership agreement was signed by all which required that henceforth voting on the hiring or release of partners arriving at the mandatory age of retirement be by written secret ballot. It also provided for waiving the restrictive clause at age sixty-two and for opportunity for confidential consultation by a partner with the "W.D.W.G." committee regarding future plans. Mr. Al Hogan who had been working with Pathology Associates was engaged as Supervisor of the Laboratory. Ralph Gamon who had been working as the Clinic's in house accountant and data processing manager was appointed Assistant Administrator and heir apparent to Arch Jenkins who had announced that he planned to retire in 1977. The surgical department decided that it needed its own coordinator and Ed Johnston was elected to fill this spot. John Platter retired to the regret of the partners but their whole hearted approval was given to his assigning his pharmacy lease to Norm Scheer who was to pay a monthly rental fee for the space he occupied. Both of these gentlemen had provided their services in an exemplary fashion and were practically members of the Clinic family. Arnold Gilstrap, the Clinic's capable maintenance man also retired this year. In March an official written notice was sent to Joe Delaney reminding him that his retirement would be effective as of June 30, 1976. After his wife's death in April he wrote to the Executive Committee requesting re-employment. This put the partners in a difficult position for although they were thoroughly sympathetic to his sad situation they felt that it was neither in Joe's nor the Clinic's best interest to grant his request. As has already been told, twenty days after his retirement he was dead.

Bill Dittman, a member of the hematology department had been spending increasing amounts of time at the hospital as a teacher and consultant. When Sacred Heart Medical Center decided that it needed a full time associate pathologist and hematologist, Bill was their choice and he decided that this was what he wanted most to do. Bill was an extremely able hematologist who loved teaching and hospital practice. In many ways the situation was similar to the one involving John Tobin over twenty years before. As with Tobin, everyone liked and respected him and wanted him happy, but not at the cost of jeopardizing the protective provisions in the partnership agreement. A committee was appointed to study the matter and recommended that the partnership agreement be revised so that a partner with fifteen years' tenure could be released without prejudice to accept a salaried position in a charitable or non-profit hospital. He would be obliged to relinquish his terminal reimbursement and agree not to carry out any fee for service medical practice or consultations for at least two years. After several months of consideration, the amendments needed to accomplish this were approved. Bill was presented with a canoe as a going away present.

As has been mentioned, during the year Jack Harrison, because of his deteriorating health requested permission to resign as a partner and continue as a salaried physician. Since this was the arrangement the partners had recommended for him in the first place and since he agreed to continue the total care of his own patients, although dropping off of the Clinic call roster, but above all since he was still at the peak of his clinical abilities and simply needed to cut back in his heretofore tremendous productivity, his request was granted.

But everyone wasn't leaving; there were a number of acquisitions to the staff this year: Dr. David E. Langdon, gastroenterologist par excellence, Dr. John F. Thaell, a hematologist and the Clinic's first Canadian, Dr. Donald D. Storey, a pulmonary specialist and Dr. Michael L. Eaton, a diagnostic radiologist. Of these only Langdon started work before the end of the year. Dave was a former Colfax boy who graduated with distinction from Washington State University and received his M.D. degree from Washington University School of Medicine in St. Louis. He interned at the University of Pennsylvania Hospital and had his residency in internal medicine at the University of California and the University of Washington. He also served a fellowship in gastro-enterology at Walter Reed Army Medical Center in Washington, D.C. He went on to a distinguished career in the United States Air Force as a flight surgeon, instructor in Aero-space medicine, internist and gastro-enterologist. Among other assignments he served as Assistant Air Attache and Physician to the Diplomatic Corps in the U.S. Embassy in Moscow, U.S.S.R. He retired as a colonel in 1975. Before coming to the Rockwood Clinic he practiced briefly in Texas where he held the position of Associate Clinical Professor of Gastro-intestinal Diseases at the University of Texas Health Science Center, Southwestern Medical School, Dallas.

Because of all the prospective additions to the staff extensive remodeling was required. The old cobalt radiotherapy area was converted into part of the diagnostic center. A new $87,000 diagnostic X-ray unit was leased and an additional office and reading room, new dressing rooms and an electrocardiographic room were added. The rent which the Clinic was paying to the Holding Corporation was increased to $15,000 a month. Surprisingly the cash position of the Holding Corporation was improved and was now in the vicinity of $28,000 in spite of the fact that three former stockholders were being paid off.

Schlicke retired as president of the Rockwood Clinic Foundation, feeling that an active member of the partnership should occupy this position. McIlvanie was elected to replace him. Its assets were now over $20,000. A grant of $3885 had been received this year from the Parke Davis Pharmaceutical Company and $2000 from the Spokane County Cancer Society.

Arch Logan was elected president of the Sacred Heart Medical Staff in May. Schlicke was now serving as president of the Pacific Coast Surgical Association. Unfortunately his wife was unable to be at his side at the meeting at which he presided the following February in Palm Springs, California since she was recovering from the prosthetic replacement of a fractured hip. At the end of 1976 Schlicke was elected chairman of the

Board of Commissioners of the Joint Commission on Accreditation of Hospitals, the governing body of the JCAH. The Joint Commission is a private, non profit voluntary organization that promotes high quality health care with optimal standards and on site surveys. Approximately 5,000 of the nation's 7,000 hospitals are accredited by JCAH. The remainder either do not seek or are denied accreditation. Recently programs have been added to accredit psychiatric hospitals, long term care facilities and ambulatory health care organizations. The JCAH was founded in 1951 as an outgrowth of the Hospital Standardization Program started by the American College of Surgeons in 1918. Schlicke had been serving on the twenty member JCAH Board as one of the three representatives of the American College of Surgeons since 1967. He had previously been on the Board of Governors of ACS for nine years and then on its policy making Board of Regents for seven years. He wound up his service to the College two years later as first vice-president.

At the end of 1976 Oeljen and Rubio were elected to become partners January 1, 1977. Rosy Hebert, the Clinic's credit manager who had been serving the Clinic in various capacities for twenty-five years was awarded a trip to visit her daughter, Sandra, in Boston. Sandra is a gifted pianist who won a $1000 National Merit Scholarship while attending Shadel Park High School. She later received musical scholarship offers from several universities but accepted the one from Boston University where she is currently working on her master's degree.

At the beginning of 1977 the "W.D.W.G." committee was directed again to study staffing and space requirements. Ralph Gamon was to start attending partnership meetings and gradually assume the duties of Business Manager in order to ensure a smooth transition when Jenkins retired in September.

There were five additions to the staff this year, three of whom had been signed up in 1976 and two new ones. Ted Thaell started in January, Mike Eaton in July, Richard G. Gower and Kenneth G Kraemer in August and Don Storey in September.

Ted Thaell was a hematologist. He attended the University of Calgary and the University of Alberta Medical School. He interned at Holy Cross Hospital in Calgary and then took a residency in internal medicine and hematology at the Mayo Clinic. He was certified by the American Board of Internal Medicine and by the Canadian Royal College of Physicians. He was an expert ice skater and played on a local amateur hockey team in Spokane.

Mike Eaton became the third member of the department of diagnostic radiology. He was a graduate of Montana State University and the University of Kansas School of Medicine. He interned at Sacred Heart Medical Center and then took a three year residency there in diagnostic radiology. Having had his post graduate training in Spokane Mike was well known to most of the Clinic staff who were most anxious to have him join them after he finished a two year stint in the Army and of course he himself had the advantage of knowing what he was walking into.

Rich Gower, an allergist and clinical immunologist, was a graduate of the University of Colorado School of Medicine. He had his internship and residency in internal medicine at the University of Miami affiliated Hospitals and then took a fellowship in allergy and immunology at the University of Colorado Medical Center.

Ken Kraemer was a hematologist and oncologist who became the fourth member of this section at the Rockwood Clinic. He received his M.D. degree from the University of Michigan and interned at the Virginia Mason Hospital. After spending two years in the U.S. Army Medical Corps he served a medical residency at the Virginia Mason Hospital and then went to the University of Washington for a two year fellowship in oncology.

Donald Storey, a pulmonary specialist, was a graduate of the University of Oregon Medical School. He had his internship and internal medicine residency at Emory University in Atlanta and then served a fellowship in thoracic disease at the Mayo Clinic.

With the rapid influx of new doctors it was suggested that the Executive Committee periodically interview new staff additions to evaluate their progress and determine their satisfaction. At about this time a medical residency was established at Sacred Heart Medical Center under the aegis of the University of Washington Medical School with Bill Dittman as the Director pro tem.

In April the American College of Surgeons in response to a request from the Chilean Chapter sent Schlicke to Santiago to discourse on the subject of hospital accreditation at the first joint meeting of the Latin American Chapters of ACS. It was a thrilling experience for him and happily soon began to bear fruit in a surge of interest and even implementation of pilot programs. He and the other guest speakers were granted an interview with President Pinochet of the Chilean Republic and were feted by the Mayor of Santiago and issued handsome certificates naming them "distinguished guests" of the capital city.

In September a farewell party was held for the Clinic's esteemed and beloved retiring Business Manager, Arch Jenkins, and he was presented with a going away gift of $5,000 a year for three years. His retirement on the thirtieth of September and subsequent departure for Hawaii left everyone with an empty feeling. It was hard to imagine the Clinic functioning without Arch but he had chosen his successor wisely and trained him well so somehow things went on. However, his absence will always be felt by those who worked with him. Friend, father confessor, superb administrator, with his sly sense of humor and his facile pen, he was unique.

It would seem highly appropriate at this point to present portions of the autobiographical "epitaph" with which he concluded his treatise "The Roots of Rockwood" since they throw light on the character of the man and his feelings about the Clinic. He says, "He [Jenkins] takes no credit for the overall growth of the medical staff, probably having been the one through the years who consistently warned about promiscuous enlargement, about growth for growth's sake, and who denied until the day he left that you grow or die,—assuming 'grow' is defined as physical and not mental.

"But he would like to be remembered as the manager who saw that his people were well trained and that his supervisors were the best obtainable. He thought it was important that patients be treated as good people with problems and would fire employees and fight doctors who thought otherwise.

"Because administration ran smoothly through the decades it is easy to overlook the fact that since 1951 the Rockwood Clinic never lost by trial or bureaucratic adjudication either a Washington State or a Federal audit of sales taxes, income taxes, wage and hour or any other rulings. Not one staff member has ever been penalized under audit for any information on a personal return which was derived from Rockwood Clinic tax returns. The Rockwood Clinic Medical Foundation is totally IRS approved as a nonprofit organization.

"He would like it remembered that the business documents and the Partnership Agreement of Rockwood are as good as they come and have been used as guidelines by many groups. Even though the possibility has been investigated by more than one sharp counselor, the documents have consistently proved to be reasonable, ethical and legal.

"Your business borrowings have been implicitly sound at good rates, your incomes have been competitive if not gargantuan.

"As he fades into the Hawaiian sunset this September of '77, the writer would urge you all to be intensely proud of the Rockwood Clinic and its place in the Inland Empire. It is the paramount outpatient medical organization in our inland part of the United States. The basic concept is good, the medical staff is superb, and—always remember—the supervisors, paramedical, and lay staff are absolutely top-rate.

"When one considers the averages for partnerships in the service field, we have had surprisingly little doctor turnover in the thirty-two years of our existence since WW II. Almost 50% of the Clinic's full time employees have been with us over three years, many over ten years....

"Furthermore, tens of thousands of patients prefer you and the Rockwood Clinic. They like the multiphasic concept. But if you want to worry about growth, look at the astounding increase in family medicine and government-backed HMOs. They are all around us. Our very same contented patients will go to them for care if they find more understanding, more available practitioners, particularly if the cost is at least as low.

"You can be the smartest bear in the forest, but if you or your organization fails to develop good doctor/patient relationships, then you can bet the average bear is going to get all the patients' huckleberries.

"What I regret is the absence of a more thorough listing of accomplishments by many of you. In some cases, the information was simply not available. I didn't have time for personal interviews. But it really isn't necessary to itemize these deeds. The patients, your peers, the community will know.

"Yet such accomplishments, whether they be medically oriented or something else done in community service, are really only microcosms, altogether adding to the reputation of the truly fine institution which is the Rockwood Clinic. Every staff member making his contribution in the manner best suited to himself and every employee having pride in where he/she works and what she/he accomplishes—this is the Rockwood Clinic."

At about the time of Arch's departure, to everyone's sorrow, Jack Harrison announced that he would no longer be able to continue the practice of medicine and would have to retire. He hoped to be able to carry on some part time work with the local Professional Standards Review Organization. The departure of this outstanding and compassionate physician was a great loss to the Clinic and a great source of distress to his patients and to the doctors who wished that there was more they could do to help alleviate his health problems. He was given a $300 retirement gift, and a search was started for a rheumatologist to replace him. Also sought were another general internist and a nephrologist.

In July of this year Arch Logan was appointed by Governor Dixie Lee Ray as the only physician on the five member Washington State Hospital Commission. This was a recent creation of the executive branch of state government to review and approve hospital revenues and budgets and set hospital rates throughout the state in the hope of helping hold down sky-rocketing health care costs. This organization was not to be confused with the Health Systems Agencies which were local bodies established under federal law to issue certificates of need to hospitals for any construction or equipment costs exceeding $150,000 of which they approved. Both agencies served only in advisory fashion with final judgement being passed by the state Department of Social and Health Services.

Rex Hoffmeister was elected president of the Northwest Rheumatism Society and president-elect of the Spokane Society of Internal Medicine. He had also been serving as a lecturer in Pharmacology at Washington State University and held a position as Clinical Assistant Professor of Medicine at the University of Washington.

The autumn brought tragedy to one Clinic family which had already had more than its share. Gayle Copsey's wife Patricia, whom everyone had loved as one of the pioneer women in the group, began having serious cardiovascular problems. Pat came from a family with a dreadful history of atherosclerosis and coronary artery disease. For some time she had been hypertensive and more recently having episodes of arrhythmia and angina. On September 8, she was hospitalized with symptoms of acute cerebrovascular insufficiency. Angiographic studies revealed almost complete atherosclerotic occlusion of her left carotid artery and Warren Peters carried out an endarterectomy. Post-operatively she developed right hemiparesis but made steady improvement after leaving the hospital.

Then, two and a half months later, just after her sixtieth birthday she was rehospitalized because of an acute episode of severe unremitting angina. Coronary arteriography revealed extensive coronary artery disease and Ralph Berg performed an aortocoronary bypass operation. Just as the operation was being completed she suffered a complete cardiovascular collapse and had to be put back on cardio-pulmonary by-pass. In spite of all efforts at resuscitation she expired on the operating table. Finch Parsons conducted the subsequent funeral service. Pat had been a fine wife and mother, an enthusiastic dancer and a great jazz buff, being in particular a devoted admirer of Duke Ellington. When Spokane's popular pianist, Arnie Carruthers, played some Ellington selections during the service there was hardly a dry eye in the house.

The partners again asked Schlicke to stay on for another year. He was pleased to accept their kind offer but stated unequivocally that he would retire in March of the next year unless a replacement was found sooner. There was considerable discussion at this time whether a fourth surgeon was really needed but upon the strong recommendation of the section of general surgery a search was started for a replacement. As it turned out an excellent replacement was found in the person of Dr. Daniel F. Cammack.

Dan Cammack grew up in a mission family in Bolivia. He was a graduate of George Fox College in Newburg, Oregon where he earned his B.A. degree. During his senior year he also took a course in medical technology at Emanuel Hospital in Portland earning his M.T. degree. As a Quaker he fulfilled his Selective Service obligations with one and a half years of service in a United States' Hospital and six months in a Friends' Mission in Peru. He was also enrolled part time in Portland State University for two years. In 1960 he entered the University of Oregon Medical School where he earned his M.D. degree. While in medical school he served externships at the Tanana Valley Clinic in Fairbanks, Alaska in the summer of 1972 and the winter of 1973. After graduation he interned at Sacred Heart Hospital in Spokane and then took a residency in general surgery at the Virginia Mason Hospital. Like Mike Eaton he knew what he was getting into when he returned to Spokane and was known and welcomed by many of the members of the Rockwood Clinic staff. However, Cammack was not available until August of 1979 so Schlicke stayed on until his arrival. It was not easy for Schlicke to make a unilateral decision about retirement, but after the Delaney debacle, although flattered by the wish of the partners for him to stay, he was anxious to have the decision his and not someone else's. After a professional life devoted to the pursuit and maintenance of high standards he was aware that his fingers were becoming arthritic and that he was not keeping up with current scientific literature as faithfully as he had in years gone by. He ardently wished to "quit while he was ahead" and before performance changes became obvious to others before they did to him.

At the last meeting of the year Langdon and Thaell were elected to partnership. This was also the year that the first of a series of illustrated feature articles concerning Clinic doctors began to appear in the Sunday supplement of the Spokesman-Review. The first was a profile of Tom Marr and told of the great job he had done over the past sixteen years organizing the Sacred Heart dialysis program and for the past twelve years officially directing the Sacred Heart Artificial Kidney Center with its home dialysis component. Later articles features Ed Johnston and his manifold interests, Sam McIlvanie and his work with transfer factor and Jon Holloway and his activities.

The holdings of the Rockwood Clinic Medical Foundation had increased to $25,600. Contributions this year included $7,000 from the Spokane County Cancer Society, $2,000 from Neil and Ellen Klemgards, Jeanne Jones $1,000 and Eric Thorn $1,000. At the annual meeting of the Foundation Trustees reports were presented on research currently being conducted and papers which had been published.

At the first partnership meeting in 1978, presumably in the spirit of a New Year's resolution one of the most futile motions on record was passed. Henceforth all staff members were to keep their offices neat and tidy or be penalized on the same basis as for delinquent paper work. Ralph Gamon announced an unbelievable collection rate approaching 99% for the preceding year. The partners met with representatives of a prepaid health plan called Northwest Health Care and later authorized individual doctors to sign up to service this plan if they wished. This was organized similar to a government funded Health Maintenance Organization (HMO) but operated by a private insurance company. To date this has worked out satisfactorily. Luther and Copsey were authorized to be out of the Clinic three or four days a month, to carry out State Industrial Insurance Examinations, the income from this service to go to the Clinic. Anxiety was expressed that because of the continued growth of the Clinic it would be increasingly difficult to obtain a unanimous vote on the admission of new members to the Partnership and a motion was made to change this requirement to a seven-eighths vote but a motion to so amend the Partnership Agreement failed. The Articles of Incorporation of the Holding Corporation were however amended increasing the capital to $200,000 (200,000 shares at $1.00) instead of the previous 100,000 shares at $1.00.

On Saturday, March 11, 1978, occurred one of the greatest, and in the minds of many, seemingly avoidable, tragedies in the history of the Rockwood Clinic. Finch Parsons had taken up flying lessons and on that day went on what was his second cross country solo flight. He had completed his student pilot flight training but was not yet qualified for instrument flying. In a rented Piper PA 28 plane he headed for Wenatchee but because of ominous weather reports decided to put down in Ephrata, where he landed uneventfully. He remained on the ground only five minutes because the weather was deteriorating rapidly and took off for his home base in Spokane. He soon encountered fog and snow flurries. The last radio message received by flight personnel at Felt's Field was that he was lost and confused. Immediately thereafter radio contact was broken off.

An extensive ground and air search was instituted but this was greatly impaired by continued bad weather. It ultimately involved over three hundred persons and 28,332 miles were logged in the air search. Five days later on Thursday, March 16, the wreckage of his green and white plane was spotted from the air. It was two thirds of the way up the side of a mountain near Hunters, Washington, just thirty-five miles northwest of Spokane. His body was identified by an Air Force "Medic" lowered to the site from a helicopter and brought out shortly thereafter. The Very Reverend Richard Coombs, Dean of the Episcopal Church of St. John where the subsequent funeral was held and who had been a great source of comfort to Finch's family during its long and trying ordeal had this to say about Finch, "He developed a remarkable ministry with patients who were terminally ill. He was the best friend I ever had....He was intelligent, mentally alert, dependable and a man of great integrity. He enjoyed life and had a great sense of humor."

His fellow radiotherapist, Don Schmutz, commented, "Many patients looked to him for emotional support, more as a priest than a physician." Finch had so much to offer everyone and for him to lose his life in his prime seemed such a waste. His death had far reaching consequences for the Clinic and was an incalculable loss to his church, his family, his profession and to his host of friends.

In keeping with previous Clinic policy regarding contributions and memorials whatever any partner wished to do out of respect and affection for Finch was left up to each individual. Due to the generosity of family and friends a beautiful stained glass window is now in the south chancel of the Cathedral in his memory. This is a Nativity scene executed by the famed Charles A. Connick stained glass firm in Boston, Massachusetts.

Finch's death placed a tremendous load on Don Schmutz in view of the heavy volume of work they had been carrying on together at Sacred Heart Medical Center so a search was instituted immediately for another radiotherapist. Larry Henry came over from Seattle on a locum tenens basis for the summer and in August Dr. David E. Davenport was signed up to join the staff later in the fall. He was a Board certified radiotherapist from Salt Lake City. He had attended the University of North Carolina and received his medical degree at the University of Utah where he also had his graduate training. Don was later presented with a bonus and granted two extra weeks of time off for his often lone heroic efforts, running the department during this trying period.

During this year two other physicians joined the staff. Dr. Thomas C. Laselle was a general internist who had graduated magna cum laude from St. John's University and had his M.D. degree from the University of Minnesota Medical School. He served his internship and residency at the Mayo Clinic. He had become well acquainted with the Rockwood Clinic while serving as Chief of Medicine at the United States Air Force Hospital at nearby Fairchild Air Force Base. Dr. Gregory L. Saue, an internist and rheumatologist, was a Dartmouth graduate. He received his M.D. degree at Temple University School of Medicine. He served a straight medical internship and residency at the University of Wisconsin Hospital and then had a fellowship in rheumatology at the University of Utah Medical Center. Board certified in internal medicine, he is board eligible in rheumatology. Arch Logan became chairman of the "W.D.W.G." committee and John Phillips replaced Stacey as medical coordinator.

On July 20, a special Partnership meeting was held to consider the resignation of Don Storey. He planned to take a teaching job at Sacred Heart Medical Center and had previously sought to embark on this course on a part time basis although still not a partner. Like other recent departures one of his first requests was that he be exempted from the provisions of the restrictive clause in the Articles of Agreement which he had signed. His request was not granted. It certainly seemed as though the Clinic was having bad luck in the pulmonary department.

A change was adopted in the Articles of Agreement this year which had previously been rejected. A candidate for partnership no longer needed unanimous approval but could be admitted as long as no more than two negative votes were cast. The partners also voted to participate in the voluntary "second opinion" program which was being organized throughout the country for the purpose of screening patients before elective surgery. They also decided to make available to the public a free blood pressure clinic to be held at the Clinic on Wednesday afternoons. This was a great success from the start although there was little demand for the second opinion option. A fiberoptic flexible sigmoidoscope was purchased to supplement Langdon's personal colonoscope for the use of which the Clinic was reimbursing him. Arthroscopy equipment was acquired for the orthopaedic department. A new xeroradiographic unit and a new electrocardiograph machine were purchased and the 12/60 autoanalyzer in the laboratory updated.

As if the conversion of the old plug-in telephone system to the new-fangled "Dimension" system in 1975 had not been hard enough on the ingrained habits of the older members, a switch was made from belt to cassette type dictating machines. Much immortal prose and many sage comments were lost to posterity when tapes were inadvertently erased or the machines not properly directed to record. The most significant investment of the year was the purchase of the Clinic's own Basic Four computer through Hubco Data Products Corporation, to be housed in remodeled space on the fourth floor.

Arch Logan reported on a recent financial appraisal of the Rockwood Holding Corporation. A re-evaluation of the stock and a reorganization of the basic structure were effected. Through the generous cooperation of the current stock-holders, stock was made available to the younger physicians at a discount rate. Almost all partners not already stockholders bought in when a reduction of the required retained earnings from $21,000 to $15,000 made money more painlessly available for purchase.

At the annual meeting of the Spokane County Medical Society in December Dick Stacey was chosen as president-elect. At the last partnership meeting of the year Dr. Scot L. Bradley, a pulmonary specialist was hired to join the staff the following year. Scot earned a B.S. degree from the University of Michigan, an M.D. from Tufts University School of Medicine and an M.S. (Medicine) from the University of Minnesota. He had his internship and residency in internal medicine at the Mayo Clinic and a two year traineeship at that institution in thoracic diseases, where he also served as an instructor and associate consultant.

Not much has been said in this history of Clinic social events, which is probably just as well since some of the first ones degenerated pretty much into brawls. The first official Christmas party was held in the old ball room on the lower floor of the old Burns mansion in which the post-war Clinic was originally located. The following year, in the hope of establishing an aura of refinement, it was held in Dr. Sharpe's home without noticeable improvement. Possibly the most riotous one of all was held a few years later at the Francis Lester. Thereafter a moratorium was declared. Finally after the move into the new building it was decided to have a decorous pre-

Christmas luncheon for the employees at the Clinic. A separate dinner party was then held, usually in the spring, for the doctors and their wives. This arrangement worked out fairly satisfactorily. It certainly saved on broken glasses and dishes but wasn't anywhere near as much fun. Various establishments in which to hold gatherings were tried through the years such as the Plantation, The Beef and Bird, the Holiday Inn and others. But as time went by and some of the more rambunctious members grew older it was felt safe once more to try a party for the whole gang. The last few years gala but eminently respectable pre-Christmas parties have been held for the doctors and the employees with assorted spouses and friends. The group had now attained a size so that it could take over the Isabella room at the Davenport Hotel or the ball room at the Ramada Inn for a buffet dinner and dancing to the music of a live orchestra. So far these have been most successful and enjoyed by all. Perhaps it was the food that made the difference.

As for educational projects, since shortly after the founding of the post-World War Two Clinic, professional scientific meetings have been held. Initially at irregular intervals, then starting in the fifties they were monthly and in recent years there have been scientific presentations on a weekly basis. Particularly interesting have been the Radiologic conferences at which current cases are reviewed and representatives of various specialties enter into the discussions.

In January, 1979, Drs. Eaton, Gower, and Kraemer became members of the Partnership. A previously formed partnership committee reported on a survey of income distribution. As a result of its findings yet another committee was appointed, particularly when it was learned that the production figures for the first quarter of the year were down from the preceding year. A patient questionnaire was developed to ascertain patient views regarding the Clinic. Because of the increased cost of performing bacteriologic studies the possibility of discontinuing this service was seriously considered. The "WDWG" committee was instructed to meet with McIlvanie and Wilson regarding their plans as they approached their sixty-fifth birthdays. The "WDWG" committee recommended changing the retirement age to seventy, the Executive Committee suggested sixty-eight but neither change was adopted by the Partnership. A motion which would require a mandatory physical examination on retiring partners who wished to continue working also failed. Dean Luther announced that he planned to retire in July of 1980 and urged that the Clinic start looking for a replacement. Ed Johnston had already announced his planned retirement in 1982 at age sixty. Contracts were ultimately signed with McIlvanie and Wilson. The former was to work full time, take his turn on the "On Call" roster and have his salary related to his production. The latter was to work mornings only except when another radiologist was away at which time he would work full time.

Due to the efforts of Tom Laselle, one half day a week specialty coverage and consultation service was established at Fairchild Air Force Base Hospital. Rich Gower became director of Internal Medicine at St. Luke's Hospital.

As the end of July approached and the time for Schlicke's final retirement drew near a delightful second retirement party was held in the penthouse on the evening of the twenty-seventh with the doctors and their wives. Several days later an afternoon party was held with the Clinic employees. That same day an emotional affair was held at Sacred Heart Medical Center. Schlicke had the feeling of imposing on his hosts as there had already been extravagant recognition of his retirement from the partnership in 1975. But in any event he was most grateful for the kindnesses shown to him and his wife. In May of 1979, at the annual Sacred Heart Medical Staff banquet he had been presented with the Sacred Heart Honor Award for Outstanding Contribution to Patient Care. This was only the second time this honor had ever been bestowed on a member of the Hospital staff. The previous recipient had been Dr. Donald G. Corbett in 1972. After Sister Peter Claver made her kind remarks in connection with the presentation she asked Schlicke, to whom this had all come as a complete surprise, if he wished to say a few words into the microphone. For once in his life he was literally speechless.

On the first of August Dan Cammack started work and Schlicke was off to a new way of life.

In December Dick Stacey was installed as president of the Spokane County Medical Society. Rex Hoffmeister was serving as president of the Spokane Society of Internal Medicine. Arch Logan was chosen as first vice governor of the Washington State Chapter ofthe American College of Physicians. Ed Johnston was still serving on the Board of Incorporators of the Medical Service Bureau and Jon Holloway as editor of the Spokane County Medical Society Bulletin. Ken Kramer had an appointment as Clinical Assistant Professor in the Department of Medicine at the University of Washington and was on the Board of Hospice Maran Atha. A number of partners had been writing some first rate scientific articles. Gayle Copsey married Louise Kemp, the widow of a prominent Spokane merchant, who among other things had been the owner of the Oxford Apartments which the Clinic now owned. Greg Saue and Tom Laselle were voted into the partnership. The Holding Corporation made a down payment on the property just north of the Clinic garages at Seventh Avenue and Bernard Street.

The Rockwood Clinic Foundation was still increasing in value. Total contributions for 1978 amounted to $13,617. The largest single private contribution was $6,800 and there were several for $1,000. Total assets were now $37,006. The Foundation minutes for this year include a letter from Ralph Gamon to CPA Schoedel assuring him that in spite of the Foundation's recent rapid growth there were no "irregularities." It was simply that because of its increased visibility due to expanded research activities and publications it was attracting more and larger donations and bequests.

As one looks back over the decade of the Seventies the continued growth and strength of the Clinic is somewhat in contrast to what was going on in the country at large. The disastrous Viet Nam War had finally drawn to a close in 1975 and student unrest on the nation's campuses had abated. The nation had weathered the Watergate scandal and the resulting resignation of President Nixon. The nation's economy was increasingly at the mercy of the oil producing countries. A recession was predicted and double digit inflation was already a fact of life. The decade ended with the deposing of the Shah of Iran and the subsequent seizure of the American Embassy in Teheran and the holding of its occupants as hostages in reprisal for the the United States having granted the Shah brief sanctuary in order to receive needed surgical and medical treatment.

Meanwhile the Rockwood Clinic was gradually moving into the computer era. Considerable automation had already taken place in the laboratory but now computers were assuming ever increasing importance in the business office. Two new stories and a penthouse had been added to the building and were being utilized. The radiotherapy department had moved its activities up to Sacred Heart Medical Center. Eighteen new physicians had been added to the Partnership. Five new salaried physicians were added to the staff, two of whom were released before the completion of the probationary period. Three partners had resigned for personal reasons and one because of poor health. These four added to the five from previous decades, two of whom had been released by the Partnership, made a total of nine over a period of thirty-four years which isn't bad for a group of this size over this length of time.

Perhaps the most significant thing which occurred at the Clinic during the Seventies was the gradual dawning of the realization that nothing was permanent and that the members of the Partnership were growing older. For so long they had regarded themselves as the bright young lights of the medical community and had lost sight of how long they had been at it. The founding partner, Bill Robinson, had long since died, Art Petersen had met with an "accidental" death, and Tom Wilder had suffered a fatal coronary occlusion, but it was not until 1974 that the first partner reached the mandatory retirement age. Thereafter three more followed during the next five years: Carl Schlicke, Sam McIlvanie and Bob Wilson. The Clinic's business manager, the operator of the pharmacy and the head maintenance man all turned in their suits. Then there was the death of Joe Delaney in 1976, and Finch Parsons fatal plane crash in 1978. Most of the members of the medical staff had devoted practically all of their professional lives to the Rockwood Clinic. They had worked hard and even made financial sacrifices at times. As a result of their efforts they now had a fine Clinic building, a staff of thirty-five doctors, and somewhere in the vicinity of one hundred and twenty-five employees. Above all they had established the legacy of a fine reputation, recognition and respect. There would seem to be no reason why, with competence, diligence, devotion and compassion, those who remain should not carry on in the same fine traditions, prosper and continue to provide high quality care to the sick and injured of this region.

THE END

Index

C

D

E

F

G

H

I

J

K

L

M

N

O

P

Q

R

S

T

U

V

W

Y

Z

THE END

COLOPHON

The Carl P. Schlicke Working Together *was printed in the workshop of one Glen Adams, which is located in the quiet country village of Fairfield, Washington, in southern Spokane County. Type for this edition was keyboarded by Miss Bobi Pearson in twelve point Baskerville type, using a Compugraphic 48 photosetter. Page numbers are in twelve point Baskerville Bold and running heads in ten point Baskerville Bold caps. The pages were printed with no enlargement of the Baskerville type. Paper stock is seventy pound Northwest Velvet. Binding is by William Bosch of Oakesdale, Washington. Camera-darkroom work is by Evelyn Foote Clausen. The sheets were printed on a 770CD Hamada offset press operated by Don Cox. Indexing is by Hilda Schlicke. The flats were stripped by Don Cox. General book design and color printing is by Glen Adams. Folding and assembly work is by Evelyn Foote Clausen. This was a fun project. We had no special difficulty with the work.*

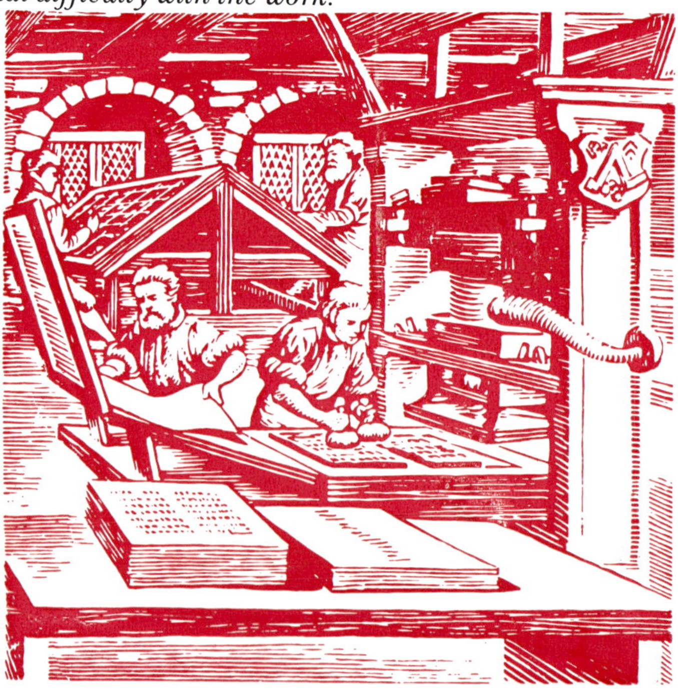